Virtual Clinical Excursions—Medical-Surgical

for

Linton:
Introduction to Medical-Surgical N

6th Edition

prepared by

Kim D. Cooper, RN, MSN
Dean, School of Nursing
Ivy Tech Community College
Terre Haute, Indiana

software developed by

Wolfsong Informatics, LLC
Tucson, Arizona

ELSEVIER
SAUNDERS

3251 Riverport Lane
Maryland Heights, Missouri 63043

VIRTUAL CLINICAL EXCURSIONS—MEDICAL-SURGICAL FOR
LINTON: INTRODUCTION TO MEDICAL-SURGICAL NURSING
SIXTH EDITION
Copyright © 2016, Elsevier Inc. All rights reserved.
Previous editions copyrighted 2012, 2007.

ISBN: 978-0-323-35869-9

Notice

Knowledge and best practice in this field are constantly changing. As new research and experience
broaden our understanding, changes in research methods, professional practices, or medical treatment may become necessary.

Practitioners and researchers must always rely on their own experience and knowledge in evaluating and using any information, methods, compounds, or experiments described herein. In using
such information or methods they should be mindful of their own safety and the safety of others,
including parties for whom they have a professional responsibility.

With respect to any drug or pharmaceutical products identified, readers are advised to check the
most current information provided (i) on procedures featured or (ii) by the manufacturer of each
product to be administered, to verify the recommended dose or formula, the method and duration
of administration, and contraindications. It is the responsibility of practitioners, relying on their
own experience and knowledge of their patients, to make diagnoses, to determine dosages and the
best treatment for each individual patient, and to take all appropriate safety precautions.

To the fullest extent of the law, neither the Publisher nor the authors, contributors, or editors,
assume any liability for any injury and/or damage to persons or property as a matter of products
liability, negligence or otherwise, or from any use or operation of any methods, products, instructions, or ideas contained in the material herein.

ISBN: 978-0-323-35869-9

Printed in the United States of America

Last digit is the print number: 9 8 7 6 5 4 3 2 1

Textbook

Adrianne Dill Linton, PhD, RN, FAAN
Professor Emeritus and Former Chair
Department of Family and Community Health Systems
The University of Texas Health Science Center at
San Antonio School of Nursing
San Antonio, Texas

Table of Contents
Virtual Clinical Excursions Workbook

Table of Contents
Linton:
Introduction to Medical-Surgical Nursing, Sixth Edition

GETTING SET UP WITH VCE ONLINE ——————————————

The product you have purchased is part of the Evolve Learning System. Please read the following information thoroughly to get started.

■ HOW TO ACCESS YOUR VCE RESOURCES ON EVOLVE

There are two ways to access your VCE Resources on Evolve:

1. If your instructor has enrolled you in your VCE Evolve Resources, you will receive an email with your registration details.

2. If your instructor has asked you to self-enroll in your VCE Evolve Resources, he or she will provide you with your Course ID (for example, 1479_jdoe73_0001). You will then need to follow the instructions at https://evolve.elsevier.com/cs/studentEnroll.html.

■ HOW TO ACCESS THE ONLINE VIRTUAL HOSPITAL

The online virtual hospital is available through the Evolve VCE Resources. There is no software to download or install: the online virtual hospital runs within your Internet browser, using a pop-up window.

■ TECHNICAL REQUIREMENTS

*   Broadband connection (DSL or cable)
*   1024 x 768 screen resolution
*   Mozilla Firefox 18.0, Internet Explorer 9.0, Google Chrome, or Safari 5 (or higher)
    Note: Pop-up blocking software/settings must be disabled.
*   Adobe Acrobat Reader
*   Additional technical requirements available at http://evolvesupport.elsevier.com

■ HOW TO ACCESS THE WORKBOOK

There are two ways to access the workbook portion of *Virtual Clinical Excursions:*

1. Print workbook
2. An electronic version of the workbook, available within the VCE Evolve Resources

■ TECHNICAL SUPPORT

Technical support for *Virtual Clinical Excursions* is available by visiting the Technical Support Center at http://evolvesupport.elsevier.com or by calling 1-800-222-9570 inside the United States and Canada.

Trademarks: Windows® and Macintosh® are registered trademarks.

A QUICK TOUR

Welcome to *Virtual Clinical Excursions—Medical-Surgical*, a virtual hospital setting in which you can work with multiple complex patient simulations and also learn to access and evaluate the information resources that are essential for high-quality patient care. The virtual hospital, Pacific View Regional Hospital, has realistic architecture and access to patient rooms, a Nurses' Station, and a Medication Room.

■ BEFORE YOU START

Make sure you have your textbook nearby when you use *Virtual Clinical Excursions*. You will want to consult topic areas in your textbook frequently while working with the virtual hospital and workbook.

■ HOW TO SIGN IN

- Enter your name on the Student Nurse identification badge.
- Now choose one of the four periods of care in which to work. In Periods of Care 1 through 3, you can actively engage in patient assessment, entry of data in the electronic patient record (EPR), and medication administration. Period of Care 4 presents the day in review. Highlight and click the appropriate period of care. (For this quick tour, choose **Period of Care 1: 0730-0815**.)
- This takes you to the Patient List screen (see the *How to Select a Patient* section below). Only the patients on the Medical-Surgical Floor are available. Note that the virtual time is provided in the box at the lower left corner of the screen (0730, because we chose Period of Care 1).

Note: If you choose to work during Period of Care 4: 1900-2000, the Patient List screen is skipped because you are not able to visit patients or administer medications during the shift. Instead, you are taken directly to the Nurses' Station, where the records of all the patients on the floor are available for your review.

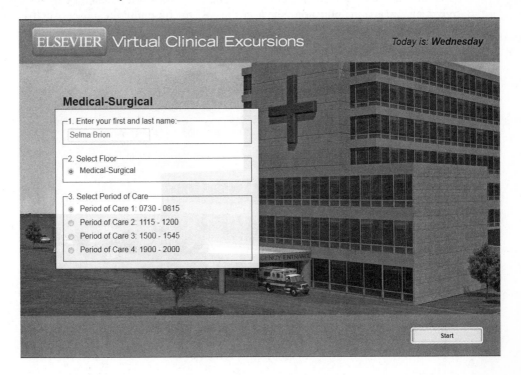

■ **PATIENT LIST**

MEDICAL-SURGICAL UNIT

Harry George (Room 401)
Osteomyelitis—A 54-year-old Caucasian male admitted from a homeless shelter with an infected leg. He has complications of type 2 diabetes mellitus, alcohol abuse, nicotine addiction, poor pain control, and complex psychosocial issues.

Jacquline Catanazaro (Room 402)
Asthma—A 45-year-old Caucasian female admitted with an acute asthma exacerbation and suspected pneumonia. She has complications of chronic schizophrenia, noncompliance with medication therapy, obesity, and herniated disc.

Piya Jordan (Room 403)
Bowel obstruction—A 68-year-old Asian female admitted with a colon mass and suspected adenocarcinoma. She undergoes a right hemicolectomy. This patient's complications include atrial fibrillation, hypokalemia, and symptoms of meperidine toxicity.

Clarence Hughes (Room 404)
Degenerative joint disease—A 73-year-old African-American male admitted for a left total knee replacement. His preparations for discharge are complicated by the development of a pulmonary embolus and the need for ongoing intravenous therapy.

Pablo Rodriguez (Room 405)
Metastatic lung carcinoma—A 71-year-old Hispanic male admitted with symptoms of dehydration and malnutrition. He has chronic pain secondary to multiple subcutaneous skin nodules and psychosocial concerns related to family issues with his approaching death.

Patricia Newman (Room 406)
Pneumonia—A 61-year-old Caucasian female admitted with worsening pulmonary function and an acute respiratory infection. Her chronic emphysema is complicated by heavy smoking, hypertension, and malnutrition. She needs access to community resources such as a smoking cessation program and meal assistance.

■ HOW TO SELECT A PATIENT

- You can choose one or more patients to work with from the Patient List by checking the box to the left of the patient name(s). For this quick tour, select Piya Jordan and Pablo Rodriguez. (In order to receive a scorecard for a patient, the patient must be selected before proceeding to the Nurses' Station.)
- Click on **Get Report** to the right of the medical records number (MRN) to view a summary of the patient's care during the 12-hour period before your arrival on the unit.
- After reviewing the report, click on **Go to Nurses' Station** in the right lower corner to begin your care. (*Note:* If you have been assigned to care for multiple patients, you can click on **Return to Patient List** to select and review the report for each additional patient before going to the Nurses' Station.)

Note: Even though the Patient List is initially skipped when you sign in to work for Period of Care 4, you can still access this screen if you wish to review the shift report for any of the patients. To do so, simply click on **Patient List** near the top left corner of the Nurses' Station (or click on the clipboard to the left of the Kardex). Then click on **Get Report** for the patient(s) whose care you are reviewing. This may be done during any period of care.

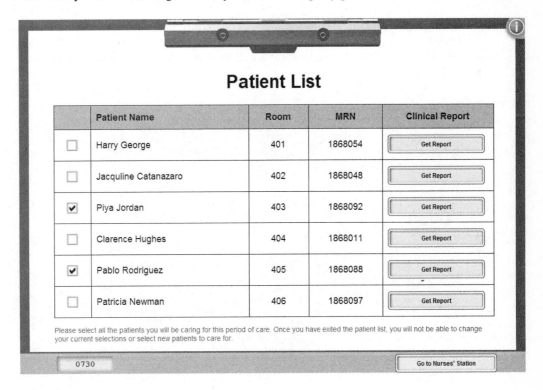

Patient List

	Patient Name	Room	MRN	Clinical Report
☐	Harry George	401	1868054	Get Report
☐	Jacquline Catanazaro	402	1868048	Get Report
☑	Piya Jordan	403	1868092	Get Report
☐	Clarence Hughes	404	1868011	Get Report
☑	Pablo Rodriguez	405	1868088	Get Report
☐	Patricia Newman	406	1868097	Get Report

Please select all the patients you will be caring for this period of care. Once you have exited the patient list, you will not be able to change your current selections or select new patients to care for.

0730   Go to Nurses' Station

■ HOW TO FIND A PATIENT'S RECORDS

Nurses' Station

Within the Nurses' Station, you will see:

1. A clipboard that contains the patient list for that floor.
2. A chart rack with patient charts labeled by room number, a notebook labeled Kardex, and a notebook labeled MAR (Medication Administration Record).
3. A desktop computer with access to the Electronic Patient Record (EPR).
4. A tool bar across the top of the screen that can also be used to access the Patient List, EPR, Chart, MAR, and Kardex. This tool bar is also accessible from each patient's room.
5. A Drug Guide containing information about the medications you are able to administer to your patients.
6. A Laboratory Guide containing normal value ranges for all laboratory tests you may come across in the virtual patient hospital.
7. A tool bar across the bottom of the screen that can be used to access the Floor Map, patient rooms, Medication Room, and Drug Guide.

As you run your cursor over an item, it will be highlighted. To select, simply click on the item. As you use these resources, you will always be able to return to the Nurses' Station by clicking on the **Return to Nurses' Station** bar located in the right lower corner of your screen.

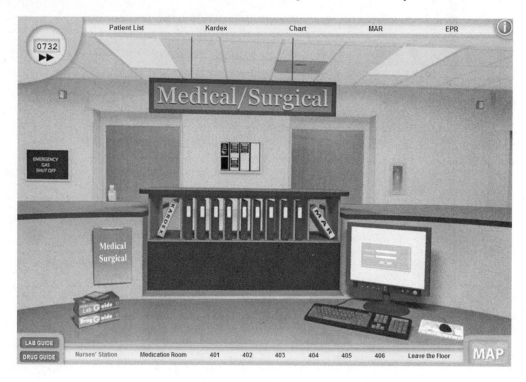

MEDICATION ADMINISTRATION RECORD (MAR)

The MAR icon located on the tool bar at the top of your screen accesses current 24-hour medications for each patient. Click on the icon and the MAR will open. (*Note:* You can also access the MAR by clicking on the MAR notebook on the far right side of the book rack in the center of the screen.) Within the MAR, tabs on the right side of the screen allow you to select patients by room number. Be careful to make sure you select the correct tab number for *your* patient rather than simply reading the first record that appears after the MAR opens. Each MAR sheet lists the following:

- Medications
- Route and dosage of each medication
- Times of administration of each medication

Note: The MAR changes each day. Expired MARs are stored in the patients' charts.

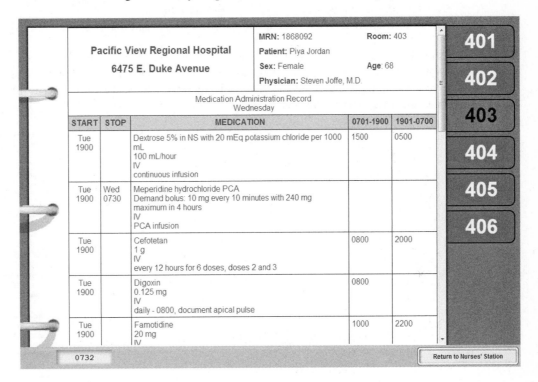

CHARTS

To access patient charts, either click on the **Chart** icon at the top of your screen or anywhere within the chart rack in the center of the Nurses' Station screen. When the close-up view appears, the individual charts are labeled by room number. To open a chart, click on the room number of the patient whose chart you wish to review. The patient's name and allergies will appear on the left side of the screen, along with a list of tabs on the right side of the screen, allowing you to view the following data:

- Allergies
- Physician's Orders
- Physician's Notes
- Nurse's Notes
- Laboratory Reports
- Diagnostic Reports
- Surgical Reports
- Consultations
- Patient Education
- History and Physical
- Nursing Admission
- Expired MARs
- Consents
- Mental Health
- Admissions
- Emergency Department

Information appears in real time. The entries are in reverse chronologic order, so use the down arrow at the right side of each chart page to scroll down to view previous entries. Flip from tab to tab to view multiple data fields or click on **Return to Nurses' Station** in the lower right corner of the screen to exit the chart.

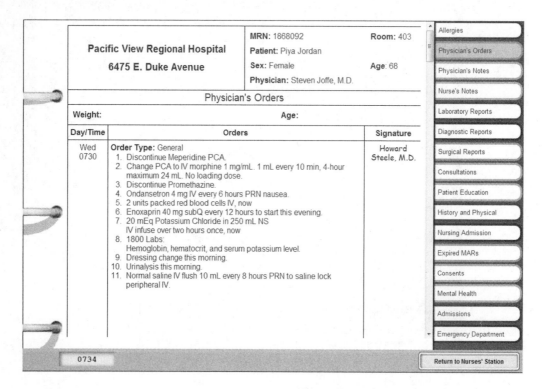

ELECTRONIC PATIENT RECORD (EPR)

The EPR can be accessed from the computer in the Nurses' Station or from the EPR icon located in the tool bar at the top of your screen. To access a patient's EPR:

- Click on either the computer screen or the **EPR** icon.
- Your username and password are automatically filled in.
- Click on **Login** to enter the EPR.
- *Note:* Like the MAR, the EPR is arranged numerically. Thus when you enter, you are initially shown the records of the patient in the lowest room number on the floor. To view the correct data for *your* patient, remember to select the correct room number, using the drop-down menu for the Patient field at the top left corner of the screen.

The EPR used in Pacific View Regional Hospital represents a composite of commercial versions being used in hospitals. You can access the EPR:

- to review existing data for a patient (by room number).
- to enter data you collect while working with a patient.

The EPR is updated daily, so no matter what day or part of a shift you are working, there will be a current EPR with the patient's data from the past days of the current hospital stay. This type of simulated EPR allows you to examine how data for different attributes have changed over time, as well as to examine data for all of a patient's attributes at a particular time. The EPR is fully functional (as it is in a real-life hospital). You can enter such data as blood pressure, breath sounds, and certain treatments. The EPR will not, however, allow you to enter data for a previous time period. Use the arrows at the bottom of the screen to move forward and backward in time.

Patient: 403 ▾   **Category:** Vital Signs ▾   **0735**

Name: Piya Jordan	Wed 0630	Wed 0700	Wed 0715	Code Meanings	
PAIN: LOCATION		OS		A	Abdomen
PAIN: RATING		5		Ar	Arm
PAIN: CHARACTERISTICS		C		B	Back
PAIN: VOCAL CUES		VC3		C	Chest
PAIN: FACIAL CUES		FC1		Ft	Foot
PAIN: BODILY CUES				H	Head
PAIN: SYSTEM CUES				Hd	Hand
PAIN: FUNCTIONAL EFFECTS				L	Left
PAIN: PREDISPOSING FACTORS				Lg	Leg
PAIN: RELIEVING FACTORS				Lw	Lower
PCA		P		N	Neck
TEMPERATURE (F)		99.6		NN	See Nurses notes
TEMPERATURE (C)				OS	Operative site
MODE OF MEASUREMENT		Ty		Or	See Physicians orders
SYSTOLIC PRESSURE		110		PN	See Progress notes
DIASTOLIC PRESSURE		70		R	Right
BP MODE OF MEASUREMENT		NIBP		Up	Upper
HEART RATE		104			
RESPIRATORY RATE		18			
SpO2 (%)		95			
BLOOD GLUCOSE					
WEIGHT					
HEIGHT					

Return to Nurses' Station

At the top of the EPR screen, you can choose patients by their room numbers. In addition, you have access to 17 different categories of patient data. To change patients or data categories, click the down arrow to the right of the room number or category.

The categories of patient data in the EPR are as follows:

- Vital Signs
- Respiratory
- Cardiovascular
- Neurologic
- Gastrointestinal
- Excretory
- Musculoskeletal
- Integumentary
- Reproductive
- Psychosocial
- Wounds and Drains
- Activity
- Hygiene and Comfort
- Safety
- Nutrition
- IV
- Intake and Output

Remember, each hospital selects its own codes. The codes used in the EPR at Pacific View Regional Hospital may be different from ones you have seen in your clinical rotations. Take some time to acquaint yourself with the codes. Within the Vital Signs category, click on any item in the left column (e.g., Pain: Characteristics). In the far-right column, you will see a list of code meanings for the possible findings and/or descriptors for that assessment area.

You will use the codes to record the data you collect as you work with patients. Click on the box in the last time column to the right of any item and wait for the code meanings applicable to that entry to appear. Select the appropriate code to describe your assessment findings and type it in the box. (*Note:* If no cursor appears within the box, click on the box again until the blue shading disappears and the blinking cursor appears.) Once the data are typed in this box, they are entered into the patient's record for this period of care only.

To leave the EPR, click on **Exit EPR** in the bottom right corner of the screen.

■ VISITING A PATIENT

From the Nurses' Station, click on the room number of the patient you wish to visit (in the tool bar at the bottom of your screen). Once you are inside the room, you will see a still photo of your patient in the top left corner. To verify that this is the correct patient, click on the **Check Armband** icon to the right of the photo. The patient's identification data will appear. If you click on **Check Allergies** (the next icon to the right), a list of the patient's allergies (if any) will replace the photo.

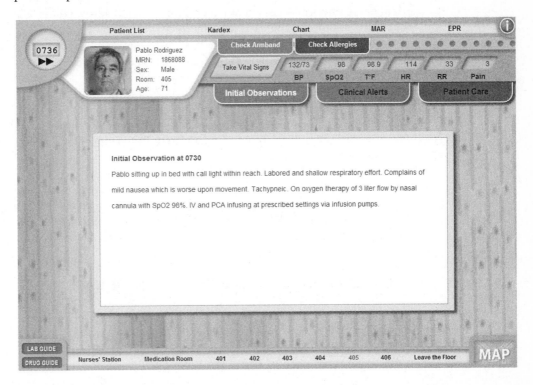

Also located in the patient's room are multiple icons you can use to assess the patient or the patient's medications. A virtual clock is provided in the upper left corner of the room to monitor your progress in real time. (*Note:* The fast-forward icon within the virtual clock will advance the time by 2-minute intervals when clicked.)

- The tool bar across the top of the screen allows you to check the **Patient List**, access the **EPR** to check or enter data, and view the patient's **Chart**, **MAR**, or **Kardex**.

- The **Take Vital Signs** icon allows you to measure the patient's up-to-the-minute blood pressure, oxygen saturation, temperature, heart rate, respiratory rate, and pain level.

- Each time you enter a patient's room, you are given an Initial Observation report to review (in the text box under the patient's photo). These notes are provided to give you a "look" at the patient as if you had just stepped into the room. You can also click on the **Initial Observations** icon to return to this box from other views within the patient's room. To the right of this icon is **Clinical Alerts**, a resource that allows you to make decisions about priority medication interventions based on emerging data collected in real time. Check this screen throughout your period of care to avoid missing critical information related to recently ordered or STAT medications.

- Clicking on **Patient Care** opens up three specific learning environments within the patient room: **Physical Assessment**, **Nurse-Client Interactions**, and **Medication Administration**.

- To perform a **Physical Assessment**, choose a body area (such as **Head & Neck**) from the column of yellow buttons. This activates a list of system subcategories for that body area (e.g., see **Sensory**, **Neurologic**, etc. in the green boxes). After you select the system you wish to evaluate, a brief description of the assessment findings will appear in a box to the right. A still photo provides a "snapshot" of how an assessment of this area might be done or what the finding might look like. For every body area, you can also click on **Equipment** on the right side of the screen.

- To the right of the Physical Assessment icon is **Nurse-Client Interactions**. Clicking on this icon will reveal the times and titles of any videos available for viewing. (*Note:* If the video you wish to see is not listed, this means you have not yet reached the correct virtual time to view that video. Check the virtual clock; you may return to access the video once its designated time has occurred—as long as you do so within the same period of care. Or you can click on the fast-forward icon within the virtual clock to advance the time by 2-minute intervals. You will then need to click again on **Patient Care** and **Nurse-Client Interactions** to refresh the screen.) To view a listed video, click on the white arrow to the right of the video title. Use the control buttons below the video to start, stop, pause, rewind, or fast-forward the action or to mute the sound.

- **Medication Administration** is the pathway that allows you to review and administer medications to a patient after you have prepared them in the Medication Room. This process is also addressed further in the *How to Prepare Medications* section below and in *Medications* in **A Detailed Tour**. For additional hands-on practice, see *Reducing Medication Errors* below **A Quick Tour** and **A Detailed Tour** in your resources.

■ HOW TO CHANGE PATIENTS OR CHANGE PERIODS OF CARE

How to Change Patients or Periods of Care: To change patients, simply click on the new patient's room number. (You cannot receive a scorecard for a new patient, however, unless you have already selected that patient on the Patient List screen.) To change to a new period of care or to restart the virtual clock, click on **Leave the Floor** and then on **Restart the Program**.

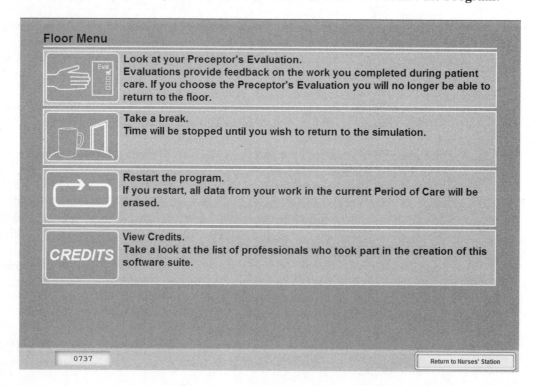

Floor Menu

Look at your Preceptor's Evaluation.
Evaluations provide feedback on the work you completed during patient care. If you choose the Preceptor's Evaluation you will no longer be able to return to the floor.

Take a break.
Time will be stopped until you wish to return to the simulation.

Restart the program.
If you restart, all data from your work in the current Period of Care will be erased.

View Credits.
CREDITS Take a look at the list of professionals who took part in the creation of this software suite.

0737

Return to Nurses' Station

■ HOW TO PREPARE MEDICATIONS

From the Nurses' Station or the patient's room, you can access the Medication Room by clicking on the icon in the tool bar at the bottom of your screen to the left of the patient room numbers.

In the Medication Room you have access to the following (from left to right):

- A preparation area is located on the counter under the cabinets. To begin the medication preparation process, click on the tray on the counter or click on the **Preparation** icon at the top of the screen. The next screen leads you through a specific sequence (called the Preparation Wizard) to prepare medications one at a time for administration to a patient. However, no medication has been selected at this time. We will do this while working with a patient in **A Detailed Tour**. To exit this screen, click on **View Medication Room**.

- To the right of the cabinets (and above the refrigerator), IV storage bins are provided. Click on the bins themselves or on the **IV Storage** icon at the top of the screen. The bins are labeled **Microinfusion**, **Small Volume**, and **Large Volume**. Click on an individual bin to see a list of its contents. If you needed to prepare an IV medication at this time, you could click on the medication and its label would appear to the right under the patient's name. (*Note:* You can **Open** and **Close** any medication label by clicking the appropriate icon.) Next, you would click **Put Medication on Tray**. If you ever change your mind or decide that you have put the incorrect medication on the tray, you can reverse your actions by highlighting the medication on the tray and then clicking **Put Medication in Bin**. Click **Close Bin** in the right bottom corner to exit. **View Medication Room** brings you back to a full view of the entire room.

- A refrigerator is located under the IV storage bins to hold any medications that must be stored below room temperature. Click on the refrigerator door or on the **Refrigerator** icon at the top of the screen. Then click on the close-up view of the door to access the medications. When you are finished, click **Close Door** and then **View Medication Room**.

- To prepare controlled substances, click the **Automated System** icon at the top of the screen or click the computer monitor located to the right of the IV storage bins. A login screen will appear; your name and password are automatically filled in. Click **Login**. Select the patient for whom you wish to access medications; then select the correct medication drawer to open (they are stored alphabetically). Click **Open Drawer**, highlight the proper medication, and choose **Put Medication on Tray**. When you are finished, click **Close Drawer** and then **View Medication Room**.

- Next to the Automated System is a set of drawers identified by patient room number. To access these, click on the drawers or on the **Unit Dosage** icon at the top of the screen. This provides a close-up view of the drawers. To open a drawer, click on the room number of the patient you are working with. Next, click on the medication you would like to prepare for the patient, and a label will appear, listing the medication strength, units, and dosage per unit. To exit, click **Close Drawer**; then click **View Medication Room**.

At any time, you can learn about a medication you wish to prepare for a patient by clicking on the **Drug** icon in the bottom left corner of the medication room screen or by clicking the **Drug Guide** book on the counter to the right of the unit dosage drawers. The **Drug Guide** provides information about the medications commonly included in nursing drug handbooks. Nutritional supplements and maintenance intravenous fluid preparations are not included. Highlight a medication in the alphabetical list; relevant information about the drug will appear in the screen below. To exit, click **Return to Medication Room**.

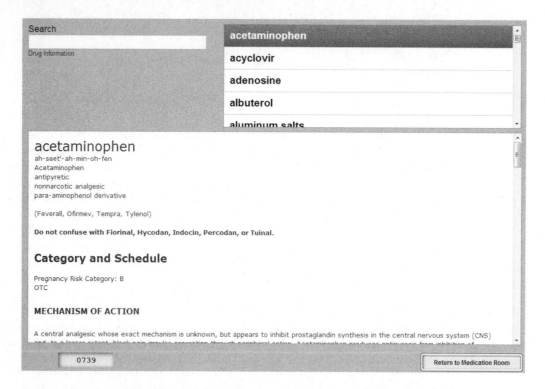

To access the MAR from the Medication Room and to review the medications ordered for a patient, click on the **MAR** icon located in the tool bar at the top of your screen and then click on the correct tab for your patient's room number. You may also click the **Review MAR** icon in the tool bar at the bottom of your screen from inside each medication storage area.

After you have chosen and prepared medications, go to the patient's room to administer them by clicking on the room number in the bottom tool bar. Inside the patient's room, click **Patient Care** and then **Medication Administration** and follow the proper administration sequence.

■ PRECEPTOR'S EVALUATIONS

When you have finished a session, click on **Leave the Floor** to go to the Floor Menu. At this point, you can click on the top icon (**Look at Your Preceptor's Evaluation**) to receive a score-card that provides feedback on the work you completed during patient care.

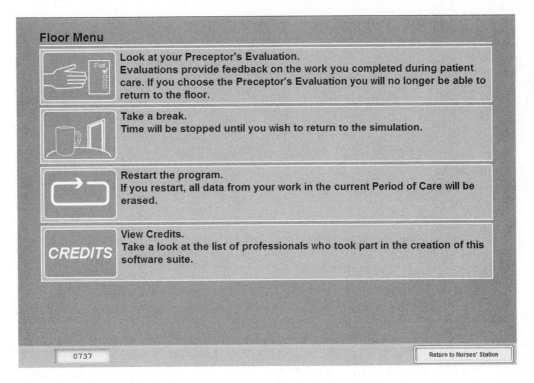

Evaluations are available for each patient you selected when you signed in for the current period of care. Click on the **Medication Scorecard** icon to see an example.

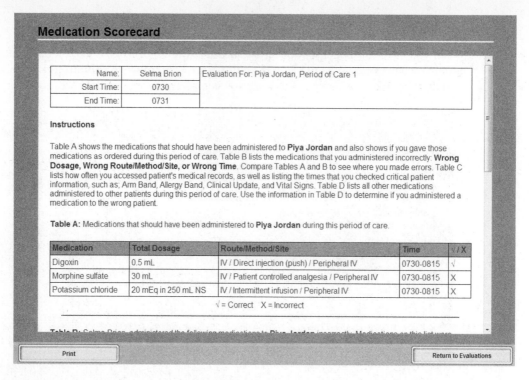

The scorecard compares the medications you administered to a patient during a period of care with what should have been administered. Table A lists the correct medications. Table B lists any medications that were administered incorrectly.

Remember, not every medication listed on the MAR should necessarily be given. For example, a patient might have an allergy to a drug that was ordered, or a medication might have been improperly transcribed to the MAR. Predetermined medication "errors" embedded within the program challenge you to exercise critical thinking skills and professional judgment when deciding to administer a medication, just as you would in a real hospital. Use all your available resources, such as the patient's chart and the MAR, to make your decision.

Table C lists the resources that were available to assist you in medication administration. It also documents whether and when you accessed these resources. For example, did you check the patient armband or perform a check of vital signs? If so, when?

You can click **Print** to get a copy of this report if needed. When you have finished reviewing the scorecard, click **Return to Evaluations** and then **Return to Menu**.

■ FLOOR MAP

To get a general sense of your location within the hospital, you can click on the **Map** icon found in the lower right corner of most of the screens in the *Virtual Clinical Excursions—Medical-Surgical* program. (*Note:* If you are following this quick tour step by step, you will need to **Restart the Program** from the Floor Menu, sign in again, and go to the Nurses' Station to access the map.) When you click the **Map** icon, a floor map appears, showing the layout of the floor you are currently on, as well as a directory of the patients and services on that floor. As you move your cursor over the directory list, the location of each room is highlighted on the map (and vice versa). The floor map can be accessed from the Nurses' Station, Medication Room, and each patient's room.

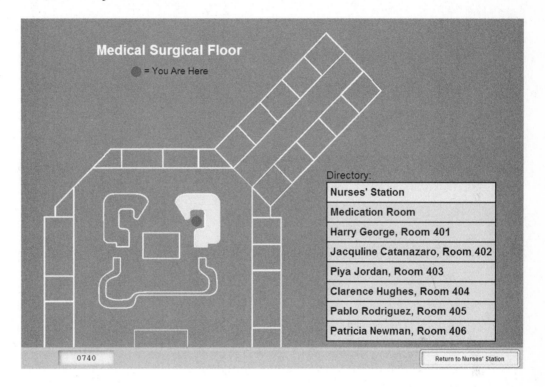

A DETAILED TOUR

If you wish to more thoroughly understand the capabilities of *Virtual Clinical Excursions—Medical-Surgical*, take a detailed tour by completing the following section. During this tour, we will work with a specific patient to introduce you to all the different components and learning opportunities available within the software.

■ WORKING WITH A PATIENT

Sign in for Period of Care 1 (0730-0815). From the Patient List, select Piya Jordan and Pablo Rodriguez; however, do not go to the Nurses' Station yet.

■ REPORT

In hospitals, when one shift ends and another begins, the outgoing nurse who attended a patient will give a verbal and sometimes a written summary of that patient's condition to the incoming nurse who will assume care for the patient. This summary is called a report and is an important source of data to provide an overview of a patient. Your first task is to get the clinical report on Piya Jordan. To do this, click **Get Report** in the far right column in this patient's row. From a brief review of this summary, identify the problems and areas of concern that you will need to address for this patient.

When you have finished noting any areas of concern, click **Go to Nurses' Station**.

■ CHARTS

You can access Piya Jordan's chart from the Nurses' Station or from the patient's room (403). From the Nurses' Station, click on the chart rack or on the **Chart** icon in the tool bar at the top of your screen. Next, click on the chart labeled **403** to open the medical record for Piya Jordan. Click on the **Emergency Department** tab to view a record of why this patient was admitted.

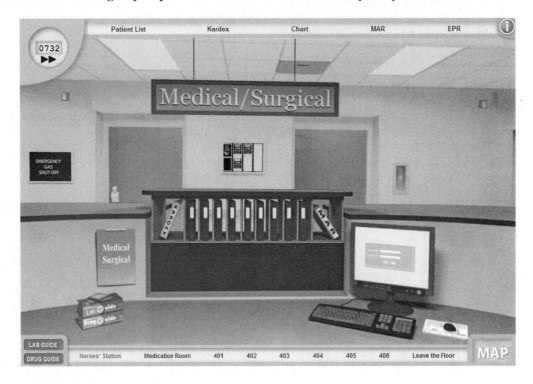

How many days has Piya Jordan been in the hospital?

What tests were done upon her arrival in the Emergency Department and why?

What was her reason for admission?

You should also click on **Diagnostic Reports** to learn what additional tests or procedures were performed and when. Finally, review the **Nursing Admission** and **History and Physical** to learn about the health history of this patient. When you are done reviewing the chart, click **Return to Nurses' Station**.

■ MEDICATIONS

Open the Medication Administration Record (MAR) by clicking on the **MAR** icon in the tool bar at the top of your screen. *Remember:* The MAR automatically opens to the first occupied room number on the floor—which is not necessarily your patient's room number! Because you need to access Piya Jordan's MAR, click on tab **403** (her room number). Always make sure you are giving the *Right Drug to the Right Patient!*

Examine the list of medications ordered for Piya Jordan. In the table below, list the medications that need to be given during this period of care (0730-0815). For each medication, note the dosage, route, and time to be given.

Time	Medication	Dosage	Route

Click on **Return to Nurses' Station**. Next, click on **403** on the bottom tool bar and then verify that you are indeed in Piya Jordan's room. Select **Clinical Alerts** (the icon to the right of Initial Observations) to check for any emerging data that might affect your medication administration priorities. Next, go to the patient's chart (click on the **Chart** icon; then click on **403**). When the chart opens, select the **Physician's Orders** tab.

Review the orders. Have any new medications been ordered? Return to the MAR (click **Return to Room 403**; then click **MAR**). Verify that any new medications have been correctly transcribed to the MAR. Mistakes are sometimes made in the transcription process in the hospital setting, and it is sound practice to double-check any new order.

Are there any patient assessments you will need to perform before administering these medications? If so, return to Room 403 and click on **Patient Care** and then **Physical Assessment** to complete those assessments before proceeding.

Now click on the **Medication Room** icon in the tool bar at the bottom of your screen to locate and prepare the medications for Piya Jordan.

In the Medication Room, you must access the medications for Piya Jordan from the specific dispensing system in which each medication is stored. Locate each medication that needs to be given in this time period and click on **Put Medication on Tray** as appropriate. (*Hint:* Look in **Unit Dosage** drawer first.) When you are finished, click on **Close Drawer** and then on **View Medication Room**. Now click on the medication tray on the counter on the left side of the medication room screen to begin preparing the medications you have selected. (*Remember:* You can also click **Preparation** in the tool bar at the top of the screen.)

In the preparation area, you should see a list of the medications you put on the tray in the previous steps. Click on the first medication and then click **Prepare**. Follow the onscreen instructions of the Preparation Wizard, providing any data requested. As an example, let's follow the preparation process for digoxin, one of the medications due to be administered to Piya Jordan during this period of care. To begin, click to select **Digoxin**; then click **Prepare**. Now work through the Preparation Wizard sequence as detailed below:

> Amount of medication in the ampule: 2 mL.
> Enter the amount of medication you will draw up into a syringe: **0.5** mL.
> Click **Next**.
> Select the patient you wish to set aside the medication for: **Room 403, Piya Jordan**.
> Click **Finish**.
> Click **Return to Medication Room**.

Follow this same basic process for the other medications due to be administered to Piya Jordan during this period of care. (*Hint:* Look in **IV Storage** and **Automated System**.)

PREPARATION WIZARD EXCEPTIONS

- Some medications in *Virtual Clinical Excursions—Medical-Surgical* are preprepared by the pharmacy (e.g., IV antibiotics) and taken to the patient room as a whole. This is common practice in most hospitals.
- Blood products are not administered by students through the *Virtual Clinical Excursions—Medical-Surgical* simulations because blood administration follows specific protocols not covered in this program.
- The *Virtual Clinical Excursions—Medical-Surgical* simulations do not allow for mixing more than one type of medication, such as regular and Lente insulins, in the same syringe. In the clinical setting, when multiple types of insulin are ordered for a patient, the regular insulin is drawn up first, followed by the longer-acting insulin. Insulin is always administered in a special unit-marked syringe.

Now return to Room 403 (click on **403** on the bottom tool bar) to administer Piya Jordan's medications.

At any time during the medication administration process, you can perform a further review of systems, take vital signs, check information contained within the chart, or verify patient identity and allergies. Inside Piya Jordan's room, click **Take Vital Signs**. (*Note:* These findings change over time to reflect the temporal changes you would find in a patient similar to Piya Jordan.)

When you have gathered all the data you need, click on **Patient Care** and then select **Medication Administration**. Any medications you prepared in the previous steps should be listed on the left side of your screen. Let's continue the administration process with the digoxin ordered for Piya Jordan. Click to highlight **Digoxin** in the list of medications. Next, click on the down arrow to the right of **Select** and choose **Administer** from the drop-down menu. This will activate the Administration Wizard. Complete the Wizard sequence as follows:

- Route: **IV**
- Method: **Direct Injection**
- Site: **Peripheral IV**
- Click **Administer to Patient** arrow.
- Would you like to document this administration in the MAR? **Yes**
- Click **Finish** arrow.

Your selections are recorded by a tracking system and evaluated on a Medication Scorecard stored under Preceptor's Evaluations. This scorecard can be viewed, printed, and given to your instructor. To access the Preceptor's Evaluations, click on **Leave the Floor**. When the Floor Menu appears, select **Look at Your Preceptor's Evaluation**. Then click on **Medication Scorecard** inside the box with Piya Jordan's name (see example on the following page).

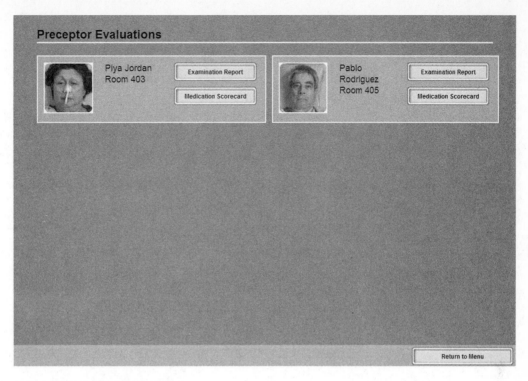

■ MEDICATION SCORECARD

- First, review Table A. Was digoxin given correctly? Did you give the other medications as ordered?
- Table B shows you which (if any) medications you gave incorrectly.
- Table C addresses the resources used for Piya Jordan. Did you access the patient's chart, MAR, EPR, or Kardex as needed to make safe medication administration decisions?
- Did you check the patient's armband to verify her identity? Did you check whether your patient had any known allergies to medications? Were vital signs taken?

When you have finished reviewing the scorecard, click **Return to Evaluations** and then **Return to Menu**.

■ **VITAL SIGNS**

Vital signs, often considered the traditional "signs of life," include body temperature, heart rate, respiratory rate, blood pressure, oxygen saturation of the blood, and pain level.

Inside Piya Jordan's room, click **Take Vital Signs**. (*Note:* If you are following this detailed tour step by step, you will need to **Restart the Program** from the Floor Menu, sign in again for Period of Care 1, and navigate to Room 403.) Collect vital signs for this patient and record them below. Note the time at which you collected each of these data. (*Remember:* You can take vital signs at any time. The data change over time to reflect the temporal changes you would find in a patient similar to Piya Jordan.)

Vital Signs	Findings/Time
Blood pressure	
O$_2$ saturation	
Temperature	
Heart rate	
Respiratory rate	
Pain rating	

After you are done, click on the **EPR** icon located in the tool bar at the top of the screen. Your username and password are automatically provided. Click on **Login** to enter the EPR. To access Piya Jordan's records, click on the down arrow next to Patient and choose her room number, **403**. Select **Vital Signs** as the category. Next, in the empty time column on the far right, record the vital signs data you just collected in Piya Jordan's room. If you need help with this process, refer to the Electronic Patient Record (EPR) section of the Quick Tour. Now compare these findings with the data you collected earlier for this patient's vital signs. Use these earlier findings to establish a baseline for each of the vital signs.

    a.   Are any of the data you collected significantly different from the baseline for a particular vital sign?

        Circle One: Yes   No

    b.   If "Yes," which data are different?

■ PHYSICAL ASSESSMENT

After you have finished examining the EPR for vital signs, click **Exit EPR** to return to Room 403. Click **Patient Care** and then **Physical Assessment**. Think about the information you received in the report at the beginning of this shift, as well as what you may have learned about this patient from the chart. Based on this, what area(s) of examination should you pay most attention to at this time? Is there any equipment you should be monitoring? Conduct a physical assessment of the body areas and systems that you consider priorities for Piya Jordan. For example, select **Head & Neck**; then click on and assess **Sensory** and **Lymphatic**. Complete any other assessment(s) you think are necessary at this time. In the following table, record the data you collected during this examination.

Area of Examination	Findings
Head & Neck Sensory	
Head & Neck Lymphatic	

After you have finished collecting these data, return to the EPR. Compare the data that were already in the record with those you just collected.

a. Are any of the data you collected significantly different from the baselines for this patient?

   Circle One: Yes   No

b. If "Yes," which data are different?

■ NURSE-CLIENT INTERACTIONS

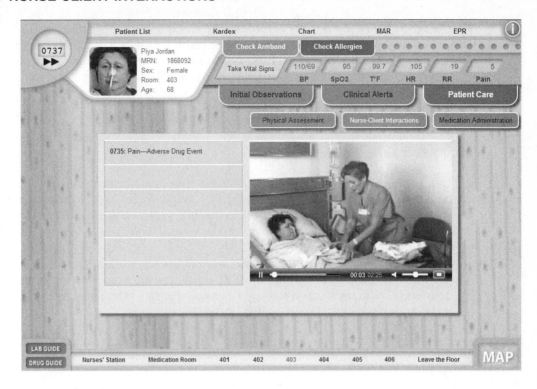

Click on **Patient Care** from inside Piya Jordan's room (403). Now click on **Nurse-Client Interactions** to access a short video titled **Pain—Adverse Drug Event**, which is available for viewing at or after 0735 (based on the virtual clock in the upper left corner of your screen; see *Note* below). To begin the video, click on the white arrow next to its title. You will observe a nurse communicating with Piya Jordan and her daughter. There are many variations of nursing practice, some exemplifying "best" practice and some not. Note whether the nurse in this interaction displays professional behavior and compassionate care. Are her words congruent with what is going on with the patient? Does this interaction "feel right" to you? If not, how would you handle this situation differently? Explain.

Note: If the video you wish to view is not listed, this means you have not yet reached the correct virtual time to view that video. Check the virtual clock; you may return to access the video once its designated time has occurred—as long as you do so within the same period of care. Or you can click on the fast-forward icon within the virtual clock to advance the time by 2-minute intervals. You will then need to click again on **Patient Care** and **Nurse-Client Interactions** to refresh the screen.

At least one Nurse-Client Interactions video is available during each period of care. Viewing these videos can help you learn more about what is occurring with a patient at a certain time and also prompt you to discern between nurse communications that are ideal and those that need improvement. Compassionate care and the ability to communicate clearly are essential components of delivering quality nursing care, and it is during your clinical time that you will begin to refine these skills.

■ **COLLECTING AND EVALUATING DATA**

Each of the activities you perform in the Patient Care environment generates a significant amount of assessment data. Remember that after you collect data, you can record your findings in the EPR. You can also review the EPR, patient's chart, videos, and MAR at any time. You will get plenty of practice collecting and then evaluating data in context of the patient's course.

Now, here's an important question for you:

> Did the previous sequence of exercises provide the most efficient way to assess Piya Jordan?

For example, you went to the patient's room to get vital signs, then back to the EPR to enter data and compare your findings with extant data. Next, you went back to the patient's room to do a physical examination, then again back to the EPR to enter and review data. If this back-and-forth process of data collection and recording seemed inefficient, remember the following:

- Plan all of your nursing activities to maximize efficiency, while at the same time optimizing the quality of patient care. (Think about what data you might need before performing certain tasks. For example, do you need to check a heart rate before administering a cardiac medication or check an IV site before starting an infusion?)

- You collect a tremendous amount of data when you work with a patient. Very few people can accurately remember all these data for more than a few minutes. Develop efficient assessment skills, and record data as soon as possible after collecting them.

- Assessment data are only the starting point for the nursing process.

Make a clear distinction between these first exercises and how you actually provide nursing care. These initial exercises were designed to involve you actively in the use of different software components. This workbook focuses on sensible practices for implementing the nursing process in ways that ensure the highest-quality care of patients.

Most important, remember that a human being changes through time, and that these changes include both the physical and psychosocial facets of a person as a living organism. Think about this for a moment. Some patients may change physically in a very short time (a patient with emerging myocardial infarction) or more slowly (a patient with a chronic illness). Patients' overall physical and psychosocial conditions may improve or deteriorate. They may have effective coping skills and familial support, or they may feel alone and full of despair. In fact, each individual is a complex mix of physical and psychosocial elements, and at least some of these elements usually change through time.

Thus it is crucial that you *DO NOT* think of the nursing process as a simple one-time, five-step procedure consisting of assessment, nursing diagnosis, planning, implementation, and evaluation. Rather, the nursing process should be utilized as a creative and systematic approach to delivering nursing care. Furthermore, because all living organisms are constantly changing, we must apply the nursing process over and over. Each time we follow the nursing process for an individual patient, we refine our understanding of that patient's physical and psychosocial conditions based on collection and analysis of many different types of data. *Virtual Clinical Excursions—Medical-Surgical* will help you develop both the creativity and the systematic approach needed to become a nurse who is equipped to deliver the highest-quality care to all patients.

REDUCING MEDICATION ERRORS

Earlier in the detailed tour, you learned the basic steps of medication preparation and administration. The following simulations will allow you to practice those skills further—with an increased emphasis on reducing medication errors by using the Medication Scorecard to evaluate your work.

Sign in to work at Pacific View Regional Hospital for Period of Care 1. (*Note:* If you are already working with another patient or during another period of care, click on **Leave the Floor** and then **Restart the Program**; then sign in.)

From the Patient List, select Clarence Hughes. Then click on **Go to Nurses' Station**. Complete the following steps to prepare and administer medications to Clarence Hughes.

- Click on **Medication Room** on the tool bar at the bottom of your screen.
- Click on **MAR** and then on tab **404** to determine medications that have been ordered for Clarence Hughes. (*Note:* You may click on **Review MAR** at any time to verify the correct medication order. Always remember to check the patient name on the MAR to make sure you have the correct patient's record. You must click on the correct room number tab within the MAR.) Click on **Return to Medication Room** after reviewing the correct MAR.
- Click on **Unit Dosage** (or on the Unit Dosage cabinet); from the close-up view, click on drawer **404**.
- Select the medications you would like to administer. After each selection, click **Put Medication on Tray**. When you are finished selecting medications, click **Close Drawer** and then **View Medication Room**.
- Click on **Automated System** (or on the Automated System unit itself). Click **Login**.
- On the next screen, specify the correct patient and drawer location.
- Select the medication you would like to administer and click on **Put Medication on Tray**. Repeat this process if you wish to administer other medications from the Automated System.
- When you are finished, click **Close Drawer** and **View Medication Room**.
- From the Medication Room, click on **Preparation** (or on the preparation tray).
- From the list of medications on your tray, highlight the correct medication to administer and click **Prepare**.
- This activates the Preparation Wizard. Supply any requested information; then click **Next**.
- Now select the correct patient to receive this medication and click **Finish**.
- Repeat the previous three steps until all medications that you want to administer are prepared.
- You can click on **Review Your Medications** and then on **Return to Medication Room** when ready. Once you are back in the Medication Room, go directly to Clarence Hughes' room by clicking on **404** at bottom of screen.
- Inside the patient's room, administer the medication, utilizing the six rights of medication administration. After you have collected the appropriate assessment data and are ready for administration, click **Patient Care** and then **Medication Administration**. Verify that the correct patient and medication(s) appear in the left-hand window. Highlight the first medication you wish to administer; then click the down arrow next to Select. From the drop-down menu, select **Administer** and complete the Administration Wizard by providing any information requested. When the Wizard stops asking for information, click **Administer to Patient**. Specify **Yes** when asked whether this administration should be recorded in the MAR. Finally, click **Finish**.

■ **SELF-EVALUATION**

Now let's see how you did during your medication administration!

- Click on **Leave the Floor** at the bottom of your screen. From the Floor Menu, select **Look at Your Preceptor's Evaluation**. Then click **Medication Scorecard**.

The following exercises will help you identify medication errors, investigate possible reasons for these errors, and reduce or prevent medication errors in the future.

1. Start by examining Table A. These are the medications you should have given to Clarence Hughes during this period of care. If each of the medications in Table A has a ✓ by it, then you made no errors. Congratulations!

If any medication has an X by it, then you made one or more medication errors.

Compare Tables A and B to determine which of the following types of errors you made: Wrong Dose, Wrong Route/Method/Site, or Wrong Time. Follow these steps:
   a. Find medications in Table A that were given incorrectly.
   b. Now see if those same medications are in Table B, which shows what you actually administered to Clarence Hughes.
   c. Comparing Tables A and B, match the Strength, Dose, Route/Method/Site, and Time for each medication you administered incorrectly.
   d. Then, using the form below, list the medications given incorrectly and mark the errors you made for each medication.

Medication	Strength	Dosage	Route	Method	Site	Time
	❑	❑	❑	❑	❑	❑
	❑	❑	❑	❑	❑	❑
	❑	❑	❑	❑	❑	❑
	❑	❑	❑	❑	❑	❑

2. To help you reduce future medication errors, consider the following list of possible reasons for errors.

- Did not check drug against MAR for correct medication, correct dose, correct patient, correct route, correct time, correct documentation.
- Did not check drug dose against MAR three times.
- Did not open the unit dose package in the patient's room.
- Did not correctly identify the patient using two identifiers.
- Did not administer the drug on time.
- Did not verify patient allergies.
- Did not check the patient's current condition or vital sign parameters.
- Did not consider why the patient would be receiving this drug.
- Did not question why the drug was in the patient's drawer.
- Did not check the physician's order and/or check with the pharmacist when there was a question about the drug or dose.
- Did not verify that no adverse effects had occurred from a previous dose.

Based on the list of possibilities you just reviewed, determine how you made each error and record the reason in the form below:

Medication	Reason for Error

3. Look again at Table B. Are there medications listed that are not in Table A? If so, you gave a medication to Clarence Hughes that he should not have received. Complete the following exercises to help you understand how such an error might have been made.

   a. Perhaps you gave a medication that was on Clarence Hughes' MAR for this period of care, without recognizing that a change had occurred in the patient's condition, which should have caused you to reconsider. Review patient records as necessary and complete the following form:

Medication	Possible Reasons Not to Give This Medication

   b. Another possibility is that you gave Clarence Hughes a medication that should have been given at a different time. Check his MAR and complete the form below to determine whether you made a Wrong Time error:

Medication	Given to Clarence Hughes at What Time	Should Have Been Given at What Time

c. Maybe you gave another patient's medication to Clarence Hughes. In this case, you made a Wrong Patient error. Check the MARs of other patients and use the form below to determine whether you made this type of error:

Medication	Given to Clarence Hughes	Should Have Been Given to

4. The Medication Scorecard provides some other interesting sources of information. For example, if there is a medication selected for Clarence Hughes but it was not given to him, there will be an X by that medication in Table A, but it will not appear in Table B. In that case, you might have given this medication to some other patient, which is another type of Wrong Patient error. To investigate further, look at Table D, which lists the medications you gave to other patients. See whether you can find any medications ordered for Clarence Hughes that were given to another patient by mistake. However, before you make any decisions, be sure to cross-check the MAR for other patients because the same medication may have been ordered for multiple patients. Use the following form to record your findings:

Medication	Should Have Been Given to Clarence Hughes	Given by Mistake to

5. Now take some time to review the medication exercises you just completed. Use the form below to create an overall analysis of what you have learned. Once again, record each of the medication errors you made, including the type of each error. Then, for each error you made, indicate specifically what you would do differently to prevent this type of error from occurring again.

Medication	Type of Error	Error Prevention Tactic

Submit this form to your instructor if required as a graded assignment, or simply use these exercises to improve your understanding of medication errors and how to reduce them.

Name: _____   Date: _____

Cultural Aspects of Nursing Care

Reading Assignment: Cultural Aspects of Nursing Care (Chapter 6)

Patients: Piya Jordan, Room 403
Clarence Hughes, Room 404
Pablo Rodriguez, Room 405

Objectives:

1. Describe cultural concepts related to nursing and health care.

2. Identify traditional health habits and beliefs of major ethnic groups in the United States.

3. Explain cultural influences on the interactions of patients and families within the health care system.

4. Discuss considerations for providing culturally sensitive nursing care.

5. Discuss ways in which planning and implementation of nursing interventions can be adapted to a patient's ethnicity.

Exercise 1

Writing Activity

30 minutes

1. Culture is defined as a patterned behavioral response that develops over time. What factors work together to shape culture?

2. Members of a _____ share values that differ from those of the dominant culture.

3. _____ nursing is the integration of culture into all aspects of nursing care.

4. _____ Although people of differing religions may have contrasting views about illness, their views concerning health are typically very similar. (True/False)

5. A patient who reports that he feels his own religious choices are best and superior to those practiced by different groups is demonstrating what behavior?
   a. Monoculturalism
   b. Ethnocentrism
   c. Stereotyping
   d. Biculturalism

6. Using both _____ and _____ communication can help reinforce the information provided to the patient.

7. When administering medications, a nurse must be aware of the influence ethnicity can have on drug therapy. Which factors could potentially affect drug therapy? Select all that apply.

   _____ Environment

   _____ Diet

   _____ Genetic differences

   _____ Nontraditional home remedies

   _____ Patient expectations

8. The beliefs of people of different ethnic groups seem to play a role in the decision of whether or not to place elders in residential facilities. The fact that the majority of residents in long-term care facilities

   are _____ _____ is evidence of these differing beliefs among cultural groups.

9. According to the "hot and cold" theory of illness, which disorders are associated with the entry of cold into the body? Select all that apply.

   _____ Dysentery

   _____ Kidney disease

   _____ Paralysis

   _____ Stomach cramps

   _____ Dental abscesses

10. Caucasians traditionally hold values related to health that include individual _____

    _____, personal _____, and _____.

11. Chinese Americans may exhibit an increased incidence of which diet-related disorders and diseases? Select all that apply.

    _____ Heart disease

    _____ Cancer of the bowel

    _____ Breast cancer

    _____ Stomach cancer

    _____ Lactose intolerance

    _____ Thalassemia deficiency

12. Members of which cultures traditionally consider touching a deceased person to be taboo?
    a. Japanese
    b. Chinese
    c. Navajo
    d. African

Exercise 2

Virtual Hospital Activity

30 minutes

- Sign in to work at Pacific View Regional Hospital for Period of Care 1. (*Note:* If you are already in the virtual hospital from a previous exercise, click on **Leave the Floor** and then on **Restart the Program** to get to the sign-in window.)
- From the Patient List, select Piya Jordan (Room 403), Clarence Hughes (Room 404), and Pablo Rodriguez (Room 405).
- For Piya Jordan, click on **Get Report**, read the shift report, and then click on **Return to Patient List**.
- Repeat the previous steps until you have read the shift report for each patient.
- Click on **Go to Nurses' Station**.
- Click **403** at the bottom of the screen and review the Initial Observations.
- Next, click on **Chart** and then on **403** to open Piya Jordan's chart.
- Click on **History and Physical** and **Nursing Admission** and review each report.
- Click on **Return to Room 403** and repeat the previous two steps with your other two patients, Clarence Hughes (Room 404) and Pablo Rodriguez (Room 405).

1. Identify the ethnic group to which each patient belongs.

   - Piya Jordan: _____

   - Clarence Hughes: _____

   - Pablo Rodriguez: _____

2. Identify the religious affiliation of each patient.

   - Piya Jordan: _____

   - Clarence Hughes: _____

   - Pablo Rodriguez: _____

3. The degree to which Piya Jordan will embrace her traditional ethnic beliefs is determined by the concept known as:
   a. cultural assimilation.
   b. ethnocentrism.
   c. cultural embracement.
   d. cultural determination.

4. Religions can be classified as Eastern or Western. Which religions are defined by the textbook as Western? Select all that apply.

_____ Buddhist

_____ American Muslim

_____ Lutheran

_____ Baptist

_____ Roman Catholic

5. Match the traditional religious beliefs/practices with the corresponding religion of Piya Jordan, Clarence Hughes, and Pablo Rodriguez.

Belief/Practice	**Religion**
_____ Importance placed on objects such as relics, statues, scapulars, and medals bearing the images of saints	a. Buddhism (Piya Jordan)
_____ May use ritual or contemplation in hopes that the last moments of consciousness may be filled with thoughts worthy of elevation to a higher existence	b. Baptist (Clarence Hughes)
_____ Belief in the need for total abstinence from alcohol	c. Catholic (Pablo Rodriguez)
_____ Belief that birth control should be limited to abstinence or natural family planning	
_____ Belief in reincarnation	

6. _____ Language may provide a source of anxiety for Piya Jordan during her hospitalization. (True/False)

7. Discuss the feelings that Piya Jordan may potentially have concerning elders.

8. Which cultures may embrace the use of healers? Select all that apply.

_____ African Americans

_____ Euro-Americans

_____ Latinos

_____ American Indians

_____ Italians

9. How do the meanings of the terms *black* and *African American* differ?

10. _____ If Clarence Hughes followed the traditional values of his culture related to illness and health, he would seek early intervention from a physician. (True/False)

11. When providing care to Clarence Hughes, the nurse must be knowledgeable about health conditions for which he is at a higher risk for developing because of his ethnic/racial background. Which diseases/disorders does Clarence Hughes have an increased risk for developing?

   _____ Diabetes

   _____ Lactose intolerance

   _____ Hypertension

   _____ Osteoporosis

   _____ Cardiovascular disease

   _____ Cirrhosis

   _____ Sickle cell disease

12. Identify at least three traditional values and/or behaviors related to health and illness that may be exhibited by Clarence Hughes within the context of his ethnic background.

13. List several beliefs about health and illness associated with Pablo Rodriguez's cultural, ethnic, and/or religious background. (*Hint:* See Table 6-1 in your textbook.)

14. In the event Pablo Rodriguez requests anointment by the hospital's priest, what can the nurse infer?
    a. He feels that he is nearing death.
    b. He feels the need to reaffirm his religious beliefs.
    c. He feels the need to confess his sins with the clergy member.
    d. He is feeling better and wishes to thank God.

Nutrition

Reading Assignment: Nutrition (Chapter 9)
Fluids and Electrolytes (Chapter 14)

Patient: Piya Jordan, Room 403

Objectives:

1. Identify the impact of fluid and electrolyte imbalances.

2. Identify age-related factors that may promote fluid and electrolyte imbalances.

3. List the functions of each of the six classes of essential nutrients.

4. Define *macronutrient* and *micronutrient*.

5. Identify the food sources of proteins, carbohydrates, and fats.

6. Identify the food sources and possible health benefits of dietary fiber.

7. Identify the food sources of each of the vitamins and minerals.

8. Describe the changes in fluid needs as an individual ages.

9. Discuss the different types of nutritional support.

Exercise 1

Writing Activity

30 minutes

1. List and describe three factors that impact digestion.

2. A patient experiencing constipation has been prescribed a diet with increased amounts of fiber. Which selection by the patient best indicates an understanding of foods that contain more fiber?
   a. Baked sweet potato
   b. Baked potato with skin
   c. Pear
   d. Corn on the cob

3. List the five major components of food.

4. Metabolic rate is largely determined by which factors? Select all that apply.

   _____ Height

   _____ Body surface area

   _____ Body weight

   _____ Race

   _____ Dietary intake

5. Which hormones are involved in the regulation of blood glucose? Select all that apply.

_____ Insulin

_____ Luteinizing hormone

_____ Thyroid hormone

_____ Epinephrine

_____ Glucocorticoids

_____ Growth hormone

6. A nurse is providing education to a patient regarding the benefits of a high-fiber diet. Which concepts should be included in the exchange of information? Select all that apply.

_____ Enhanced bowel functioning

_____ Increased energy

_____ Reduced blood cholesterol

_____ Increased rate of glucose absorption

_____ Reduced incidence of colon cancer development

7. A patient has been advised to increase her intake of folic acid in preparation for pregnancy. Which foods should be included in this plan? Select all that apply.

_____ Milk

_____ Eggs

_____ Dried beans

_____ Whole grain products

_____ Yeast

_____ Wheat germ

_____ Leafy green vegetables

8. A patient who has been instructed to begin taking a multivitamin supplement daily questions why this is necessary. Which statement regarding vitamins is correct?
   a. Vitamins are organic substances.
   b. Vitamins provide energy.
   c. Water-soluble vitamins include the B complexes and vitamin C.
   d. Fat-soluble vitamins cannot be stored in the body.

9. Major minerals are responsible for enzyme regulation, _____ balance, osmotic

   pressure, and maintenance of nerve and muscle _____.

10. A nurse is providing care for a patient suspected of being malnourished. Which diagnostic test will provide the best information to confirm these suspicions?
    a. Serum albumin
    b. Urinalysis
    c. Hematocrit (Hct)
    d. Complete blood count (CBC)

11. A diet high in fat has been associated with the development of _____

    _____, _____, and _____.

12. While being seen at the physician's office for a routine physical examination, a patient tells a nurse that he has been hearing a great deal of "hype" about antioxidants. He asks the nurse to explain what they are. Which statement about antioxidants is most accurate?
    a. Antioxidants are plant pigments found in yellow fruits and vegetables.
    b. Antioxidants are hormone-like substances found in whole grains and legumes.
    c. Antioxidants are contained in some foods and are believed to have a role in the Prevention of cancer.
    d. Antioxidants are proteins found in onions and wines that are linked to a reduction in the risk for diabetes.

13. A patient attempting to follow a healthy diet asks about the amount of whole grains needed each day. Which is the best response to give to this patient?
    a. "You should try to eat at least 3 ounces of whole grains each day."
    b. "You should eat no more than 4 ounces of whole grains each day."
    c. "You should eat between 2 and 3 ounces of whole grains each day."
    d. "There is no current differentiation between grains and whole grains."

14. Which are potential complications associated with enteral tube feedings? Select all that apply.

    _____ Hunger

    _____ Vomiting

    _____ Hyperkalemia

    _____ Hypernatremia

    _____ Diarrhea

Exercise 2

Virtual Hospital Activity

45 minutes

- Sign in to work at Pacific View Regional Hospital for Period of Care 2. (*Note:* If you are already in the virtual hospital from a previous exercise, click on **Leave the Floor** and then on **Restart the Program** to get to the sign-in window.)
- From the Patient List, select Piya Jordan (Room 403).
- Click on **Get Report** and read the shift report.
- Click on **Go to Nurses' Station**.
- Click on **Chart** and then on **403** to view Piya Jordan's chart.
- Click on and review the **History and Physical** and **Nursing Admission**.

1. What is Piya Jordan's chief complaint at the time of admission?

2. For how long have Piya Jordan's symptoms persisted?

3. Piya Jordan's weight is _____ pounds (_____ kilograms), and she is _____ inches tall.

4. Piya Jordan reports a recent weight loss of _____ pounds.

5. Review Piya Jordan's weight loss and current weight. This weight loss is considered to be which classification?
   a. Mild
   b. Moderate
   c. Severe

6. Based on her age and sedentary lifestyle, how many calories per day does Piya Jordan require?
   a. 1200
   b. 1500
   c. 1600
   d. 2200

• Click on and review the **Laboratory Reports** in Piya Jordan's chart.

7. Piya Jordan's hematocrit levels range between _____% and _____%.

8. Normal hematocrit levels for women are between _____% and _____%.

9. Which statements concerning hematocrit levels are correct? Select all that apply.

   _____ Hematocrit levels indicate the amount of protein in the body.

   _____ Hematocrit levels indicate the amount of iron in the body.

   _____ Hematocrit levels are the same for both men and women.

   _____ Hematocrit levels can be altered as a result of a surgical intervention.

   _____ Decreased hematocrit levels are associated with dehydration.

10. Urine specific gravity is normally between _____ and _____.

11. Piya Jordan's urine specific gravity is _____.

12. Indicate whether each statement is true or false.

    a. _____ A reduced urine specific gravity is indicative of hypovolemia.

    b. _____ Based on a review of Piya Jordan's laboratory findings, the mean corpuscular volume (MCV) indicates the presence of anemia.

- Click on and review the **Physician's Notes** and **Physician's Orders**.

13. Which events can increase the body's nutritional needs? Select all that apply.

    _____ Infection

    _____ Fever

    _____ Trauma

    _____ Stress

    _____ Rest

14. Piya Jordan's cancer places her at risk for which nutrition-related complications? Select all that apply.

    _____ Protein deficiency

    _____ Positive nitrogen balance

    _____ Negative nitrogen balance

    _____ Hyperbilirubinemia

    _____ Hypercalcemia

15. What diet has been ordered for Piya Jordan?

16. What nutrition is being provided to Piya Jordan during this stage of her recovery?

17. Considering Piya Jordan's age, how much fluid is needed per kilogram of body weight?
    a. 15 mL/kg
    b. 20 mL/kg
    c. 25 mL/kg
    d. 30 mL/kg

18. Over the course of a 24-hour day, Piya Jordan will receive _____ mL of the 5% dextrose in normal saline (D_5NS) infusion.

19. Piya Jordan is 68 years old. What age-related changes increase her risk for fluid and electrolyte imbalances?

20. Which best describes Piya Jordan's prescribed intravenous fluids?
    a. A Ringer's solution
    b. A source of total parenteral nutrition
    c. A hypotonic dextrose solution
    d. An isotonic saline solution
    e. A hypertonic dextrose solution

21. Which statement best explains the intended action of Piya Jordan's ordered intravenous solution (D_5NS)?
    a. The solution mimics electrolyte concentration of blood.
    b. The solution is often used as a volume expander.
    c. The solution provides energy and nutrients for cellular function and repair.
    d. The solution expands extracellular fluid without changing osmolality.

22. Piya Jordan's IV site must be assessed frequently. The presence of complications can be identified by manifestations at the site and by observations of the patient. Match each of the complications below with the corresponding clinical manifestation.

Complication	Clinical Manifestation
_____ Infiltration	a. Heat, pain, redness, and edema
_____ Phlebitis	b. Heat, pain, redness, edema, and possible fever and sepsis
_____ Infection	c. Fluid that will not flow by gravity; site that is edematous, blanched, painful, and cold
_____ Air embolism	d. Rash, redness, and itching
_____ Allergic reaction	e. Cyanosis, tachycardia, and decreased blood pressure
_____ Circulatory overload	f. Dyspnea, cough, cyanosis, and jugular vein distention

23. After _____ days without oral nutrition, enteral methods may be indicated.

24. A nasogastric (NG) tube may be used for which reasons? Select all that apply.

_____ Decompression—removal of secretions and gases from the GI tract

_____ Feeding—instillation of liquid supplements or feedings into the stomach

_____ Compression—internal application of pressure by means of an inflated balloon to prevent internal GI hemorrhage

_____ Evacuation—reduction of intestinal stool contents

_____ Lavage—irrigation of stomach; used in cases of active bleeding, poisoning, or gastric dilation

25. A nurse is planning to clean Piya Jordan's nostril where the NG tube has been placed. Which solution is most appropriate to use for this intervention?
    a. Alcohol-based solution
    b. Mild soap and water
    c. Hydrogen peroxide
    d. Water-soluble lubricant

26. When monitoring Piya Jordan's NG output, which findings may indicate fluid volume deficits? Select all that apply.

_____ Hypotension

_____ Pulse of more than 20 beats/minute above the baseline values

_____ Hypertension

_____ Urine production of less than 50 mL/hour for 2 or more consecutive hours

_____ Confusion

27. Output totals of _____ mL or greater from the NG tube warrant notification of the physician.

28. Use the guidelines from My Daily Food Plan to match each food group with the recommended daily serving size.

Food Group	Recommended Daily Serving
_____ Grains	a. 3 cups per day
_____ Vegetables	b. 6 ounces per day
_____ Fruits	c. 5.5 ounces per day
_____ Dairy	d. 2.5 cups per day
_____ Protein foods	e. 2 cups per day

Developmental Processes and the Older Adult

Reading Assignment: Developmental Processes (Chapter 10)
The Older Patient (Chapter 11)

Patient: Clarence Hughes, Room 404

Objectives:

1. List the developmental tasks for successful adulthood.

2. Identify the health problems specific to the adult age groups.

3. Discuss the health care needs of young, middle, and older adults.

4. Describe modifications needed for activities of daily living.

5. Determine the extent to which selected myths and stereotypes about older adults are factual.

6. Describe biologic, physiologic, and psychosocial factors associated with aging.

7. Explain why drug adjustments may be needed for older persons.

Exercise 1

Writing Activity

30 minutes

1. Identify the developmental tasks that must be achieved by young adults. Select all that apply.

   _____ Discover new satisfaction with a mate or significant other

   _____ Begin preparation for retirement

   _____ Establish independence

   _____ Become established in a vocation or profession that provides personal satisfaction, economic independence, and a feeling of making a worthwhile contribution

   _____ Maintain a home and manage a time schedule and life stresses

2. The physiologic development of a living being and the qualitative changes seen in the body are known

   as _____.

3. _____ is the progression of behavioral changes that involve the acquisition of appropriate cognitive, linguistic, and psychosocial skills.

4. The study of aging is known as _____.

5. _____ is a stereotype, prejudice, or discrimination against people, especially older adults, based on their age.

6. _____ Some degree of intellectual decline is a normal part of aging. (True/False)

7. Identify the stages of adulthood and include the age range for each stage.

8. A student nurse is preparing a presentation concerning the "sandwich generation." Which statement about this concept is correct?
   a. The name is derived from the amount of fast food consumed during this stage of development.
   b. Members of the sandwich generation include school-age children.
   c. Adults in their middle years are members of this category.
   d. Older adults are members of the sandwich generation.

9. If a nurse is performing an assessment on a middle adult patient, which must be included to determine successful completion of the appropriate developmental tasks?
    a. Assess for the presence of meaningful, intimate relationships
    b. Assess for signs of depression, such as excessive sleeping and decreased appetite
    c. Ask the patient if he or she feels lonely
    d. Assess for the presence of parental support systems

10. What is the major cause of death for patients between the ages of 39 and 45?
    a. Suicide
    b. Homicide
    c. Cancer
    d. Accidents

11. A middle-age female patient asks about her risk for osteoporosis during this period in her life. Which is the best response by the nurse?
    a. "Osteoporosis is not a concern until late adulthood."
    b. "Osteoporosis is only an issue for underweight women."
    c. "Osteoporosis is a greater concern for young women of childbearing age."
    d. "It is too late to prevent osteoporosis-related complications."
    e. "Osteoporosis is a concern for women in middle age."

12. What is the leading cause of death for the older adult?
    a. Heart disease
    b. Unintentional injuries
    c. Acquired immunodeficiency syndrome (AIDS)
    d. Bone cancer

13. Which refers to the functional capabilities of various organ systems in the body?
    a. Biologic age
    b. Psychologic age
    c. Social age
    d. Chronologic age

14. When providing health education to a preteen female, the nurse should incorporate which statement into the teaching?
    a. The rate of physical growth exceeds the rate of cognitive development.
    b. If the child had begun to demonstrate physical changes, she is considered to be an adolescent.
    c. Some girls in this age group may begin to demonstrate the changes associated with puberty.
    d. The rate of physical growth exceeds the rate of psychosocial development.

Exercise 2

Virtual Hospital Activity

30 minutes

- Sign in to work at Pacific View Regional Hospital for Period Care 2. (*Note:* If you are already in the virtual hospital from a previous exercise, click on **Leave the Floor** and then on **Restart the Program** to get to the sign-in window.)
- From the Patient List, select Clarence Hughes (Room 404).
- Click on **Get Report** and read the shift report.
- Click on **Go to Nurses' Station**.
- Click on **404** at the bottom of the screen to enter the patient's room.
- Click on **Check Armband** and then on **Take Vital Signs**. Review the information given.

1. How old is Clarence Hughes?

2. In what phase of adulthood is Clarence Hughes?

3. Which Erikson stage of development is applicable to Clarence Hughes?
   a. Trust vs. mistrust
   b. Ego integrity vs. despair
   c. Generativity vs. stagnation
   d. Identity vs. identity confusion

4. Which are developmental tasks that Clarence Hughes must face during this phase of his life? Select all that apply.

   _____ Reflection on one's own mortality

   _____ Interest in community activities

   _____ Longing to participate in civic matters

   _____ Acceptance of one's own death

   _____ Begin to share duties with one's life partner

- Click on **Chart** and then on **404**.
- Click on and review the **Nursing Admission**.

5. Why has Clarence Hughes been admitted to the hospital?

- Click on and review the **History and Physical**.

6. Which items from Clarence Hughes' personal history can be associated with aging? Select all that apply.

_____ Osteoarthritis

_____ Glaucoma

_____ Degenerative joint disease

_____ Slight prostrate enlargement

_____ History of appendectomy

- Click on **Return to Room 404**.
- Click on **Patient Care** and then on **Physical Assessment**.
- Complete a head-to-toe assessment by clicking on the body system categories (yellow buttons) and body system subcategories (green buttons).

7. What, if any, age-related changes are noted in Clarence Hughes' physical assessment?

- Click on **MAR** and then on tab **404**.
- Review the medications ordered for Clarence Hughes.

8. Which statements concerning the use of medications in older adults are true? Select all that apply.

_____ On average, the older adult takes up to seven prescription medications.

_____ Laxatives and vitamin supplements are commonly used medications among older adults.

_____ The average older adult is currently taking only two prescription medications.

_____ The use of multiple drugs will enhance the therapeutic benefits of the medications taken.

_____ Using more than one pharmacy to fill prescriptions will increase risk factors associated with polypharmacy.

_____ The body's ability to absorb, transport, and eliminate medications is increased with age.

• Click on **Return to Room 404**.
• Click on the **Drug** icon in the lower left corner.
• Review the information for each of the medications ordered for Clarence Hughes.

9. The medications listed below have been prescribed for Clarence Hughes. Which of the medications have special life span considerations listed for older adults? Select all that apply.

_____ Celecoxib

_____ Timolol maleate

_____ Docusate sodium

_____ Pilocarpine 1% ophthalmic solution

_____ Enoxaparin

_____ Promethazine hydrochloride

_____ Magnesium hydroxide

_____ Aluminum hydroxide with magnesium and simethicone

_____ Bisacodyl

10. Which are manifestations associated with adverse drug reactions in the older adult? Select all that apply.

_____ Restlessness

_____ Falls

_____ Excitability

_____ Depression

_____ Altered mental states

_____ Diarrhea

_____ Urinary incontinence

11. Match each drug classification with the corresponding age-related adverse reaction.

Drug Classification	Adverse Reaction
_____ Antibiotics	a. Drowsiness
_____ Antidepressants	b. Nephrotoxicity
_____ Antipsychotics	c. Confusion
_____ Diuretics	d. Hypokalemia
_____ Sedatives/hypnotics	e. Sedation

12. Identify several factors that can reduce medication-related complications in the older adult patient.

Inflammation, Infection, and Immunity

Reading Assignment: Nutrition (Chapter 9)
Immunity, Inflammation, and Infection (Chapter 13)
Immunologic Disorders (Chapter 34)

Patient: Harry George, Room 401

Objectives:

1. Describe physical and chemical barriers to infection.

2. Describe how inflammatory changes act as bodily defense mechanisms.

3. Identify the signs and symptoms of inflammation.

4. Discuss the process of repair and healing.

5. Differentiate between infection and inflammation.

6. Describe the ways that infections are transmitted.

7. Identify the signs and symptoms of infection.

8. Compare community-acquired and health care-associated infections.

9. Discuss the nursing care of patients with infections.

Exercise 1

Writing Activity

20 minutes

1. The body's first lines of defense are the _____ and _____

   _____.

2. Match each cell type with the corresponding role in immunity.

   Cell Type

   _____ Neutrophils

   _____ Monocytes

   _____ Eosinophils

   _____ Basophils

   _____ B lymphocytes

   _____ T lymphocytes

   Role

   a. Increase the body's immune response

   b. Fight bacterial infections

   c. Initiate the inflammatory response and release histamine

   d. Produce antibodies

   e. Ingest foreign antigens

   f. Fight parasitic infections and demonstrate an increase during allergic reactions

3. Match each action of the inflammatory process with the corresponding order of occurrence.

   Action

   _____ Chemical mediation

   _____ Hemodynamic change

   _____ Antiinflammation hormones released

   _____ Increased capillary permeability

   Order of Occurrence

   a. First

   b. Second

   c. Third

   d. Fourth

4. A patient has been diagnosed with ringworm infection. This infection is best characterized as which type?
   a. Viral infection
   b. Bacterial infection
   c. Protozoan infection
   d. Fungal infection

5. By which mode of contact is a sexually transmitted disease transferred?
   a. Direct contact
   b. Indirect contact
   c. Multifocal contact
   d. Common vehicle transmission

6. A nurse working in a physician's office should recognize that which diseases and/or infections are considered reportable? Select all that apply.

    _____ Herpes simplex

    _____ Gonorrhea

    _____ Candidiasis

    _____ Rubella

    _____ Tetanus

7. _____-_____ infections are acquired in day-to-day contact with the public.

8. What term is used to refer to hospital-acquired infections? Please include both the former term and the current term.

9. The nurse is caring for a a patient being treated for an iatrogenic infection. Which statement by the patient indicates an understanding of the condition?
    a. "Antibiotics will not adequately manage this disorder."
    b. "This infection is best treated with antiviral medications."
    c. "Isolation practices will be vital to managing my condition."
    d. "My disorder is the result of treatments for another disorder."

10. Match each disorder with the correct method of precaution that should be put in place in order to prevent transmission. (*Note:* Some methods will be used more than once.)

Disease	**Method of Precaution**
_____ Measles	a. Airborne precautions
_____ Varicella	b. Droplet precautions
_____ Mumps	c. Contact precautions
_____ Tuberculosis	
_____ *Clostridium difficile* infection	
_____ Scabies	
_____ Pediculosis	
_____ Influenza	

11. Discuss the difference between antigens and antibodies.

Exercise 2

Virtual Hospital Activity

45 minutes

- Sign in to work at Pacific View Regional Hospital for Period of Care 1. (*Note:* If you are already in the virtual hospital from a previous exercise, click on **Leave the Floor** and then on **Restart the Program** to get to the sign-in window.)
- From the Patient List, select Harry George (Room 401).
- Click on **Get Report** and read the shift report.
- Click on **Go to Nurses' Station**.
- Click on **Chart** and then on **401**.
- Click on and review the **Nursing Admission** and **History and Physical**.

1. What were Harry George's chief complaints upon arrival to the Emergency Department?

2. What medical diagnoses are listed on the History and Physical?

- Click on and review the **Laboratory Reports**.

3. How is Harry George's infection best classified?
   a. Viral
   b. Bacterial
   c. Fungal
   d. Parasitic

4. The physician has ordered an erythrocyte sedimentation rate (ESR). Which statement best describes this test?
   a. The ESR is suppressed in the presence of inflammation.
   b. An infectious process will reduce the ESR.
   c. The ESR is elevated in the presence of inflammation.
   d. The ESR is naturally suppressed in alcohol-dependent patients.

5. Which tests will be ordered to confirm the presence of the infection in Harry George? Select all that apply.

   _____ Complete blood count (CBC)

   _____ Culture and sensitivity of wound

   _____ Urinalysis

   _____ Magnetic resonance imaging (MRI)

   _____ Folic acid level

   _____ Blood alcohol level

6. Harry George's white blood cell (WBC) count has ranged from _____ on Monday to

   _____ on Tuesday.

7. What is the normal range for the white blood cell count?
   a. 2,000-4,500
   b. 4,000-7,500
   c. 5,000-10,000
   d. 10,000-12,000

8. The pathogen identified as the causative agent in Harry George's infection is

   _____ _____.

9. The causative agent in Harry George's infection can be further identified as:
   a. bacterial.
   b. fungal.
   c. protozoan.
   d. rickettsiae.
   e. parasitic.

- Click on **Return to Nurses' Station** and then on **401** at the bottom of the screen.
- Review the Initial Observations.
- Click on **Patient Care** and then on **Physical Assessment**.
- Complete a head-to-toe systems assessment by clicking on the body system categories (yellow buttons) and body system subcategories (green buttons).

10. What findings in Harry George's lower extremities support the presence of an infection?

11. _____ It is a legal requirement that Harry George's infection be reported to the appropriate public health officials. (True/False)

12. When the nurse is preparing to care for Harry George, which precaution is warranted?
    a. Enteric precautions
    b. Droplet precautions
    c. Reverse isolation
    d. Airborne precautions
    e. Standard precautions
    f. Universal precautions

13. What places Harry George at the greatest risk for developing a health care-associated infection?
    a. Indwelling Foley catheter
    b. Increasing pain
    c. History of alcohol abuse
    d. Homelessness

14. Which stage of the antiinflammatory response is most likely being found in Harry George's assessment?
    a. Stage 1
    b. Stage 2
    c. Stage 3
    d. Stage 4

15. Harry George's wound has redness, warmth, and swelling. This is representative of the

    _____ changes in the inflammatory process.

- Click on **MAR** and then on **401**.
- Review Harry George's ordered medications. (*Hint:* If necessary, refer to the Drug Guide for assistance.)

16. What medications have been ordered to manage Harry George's infection?

17. Which assessments related to Harry George's IV therapy are indicated as a result of the prescribed gentamicin? Select all that apply.

_____   Induration

_____   Heat along vein

_____   Redness surrounding IV site

_____   Presence of red streaks

_____   Pain

18. Which manifestation is consistent with a serious complication of the administration of gentamicin?
    a. Nausea
    b. Genital pruritus
    c. Lethargy
    d. Diarrhea

19. When assisting Harry George to select his meals, which should be encouraged to promote wound healing?
    a. Citrus fruits
    b. Dairy products
    c. Whole grains
    d. Eggs

Pain Management

Reading Assignment: Pain Management (Chapter 15)

Patients: Harry George, Room 401
Pablo Rodriguez, Room 405

Objectives:

1. Define *pain*.

2. Explain the physiologic basis for pain.

3. Identify situations in which patients are likely to experience pain.

4. Explain the relationships between a patient's pain and past pain experiences, anticipation, culture, anxiety, and/or activity.

5. Identify differences in the duration of acute and chronic pain and discuss patient responses to each.

6. Explain the special needs of the older adult patient with pain.

7. List the data to be collected when assessing pain.

8. Describe the nursing care of patients receiving opioid and nonopioid analgesics for pain.

9. List the factors that should be considered when pain is not relieved with analgesic medications.

Exercise 1

Writing Activity

30 minutes

1. _____ are pain receptors located in the muscles, tendons, subcutaneous tissue, and the skin.

2. _____ are the body's natural opioid-like substances that block the transmission of painful impulses to the brain.

3. A _____ is an inactive substance used in research or clinical practice to determine the effects of a legitimate drug or treatment.

4. Which are factors that can increase the body's endorphin levels? Select all that apply.

   _____ Age

   _____ Gender

   _____ Brief stress

   _____ Pain

   _____ Laughter

   _____ Exercise

   _____ Beliefs about pain

5. Identify several physical factors that can affect a patient's perception of pain.

6. Indicate whether each statement is true or false.

   a. _____ Gender can affect an individual's pain threshold and tolerance.

   b. _____ While caring for a patient who has recently been medicated for complaints of pain, it is appropriate for the patient's nurse to ask a nursing assistant to recheck the patient's level of pain.

7. A nurse is planning to use heat to manage a patient's pain. Which statements concerning the use of heat therapy are correct? Select all that apply.

_____ Heat therapy may be alternated with cold therapy.

_____ Heat therapy is contraindicated in patients with peripheral vascular disease.

_____ Heat therapy should be limited to 30 minutes per application.

_____ Heat applications may be moist or dry.

_____ Heat is a safe, effective means to manage pain related to a malignant tumor.

8. A nurse is preparing to provide an inservice on the use of alternative treatments for pain. Which concepts are correct and may be included in the presentation? Select all that apply.

_____ Chiropractic treatments may increase patient depression.

_____ Massage therapy may lessen anxiety and depression.

_____ Music therapy has no untoward side effects.

_____ Unwillingness to be touched may hinder the success of massage therapy.

_____ Music therapy is an expensive alternative for pain management.

9. A _____ unit involves the application of external electrical stimulation of the skin and underlying tissues through electrodes attached to the skin.

10. While caring for a patient, a nurse notes the presence of agitation, insomnia, diarrhea, and sweating after requests for "stronger" analgesics are refused by the physician. What is being demonstrated by the patient?
    a. The patient has developed a tolerance to all analgesics.
    b. The patient has developed psychologic dependence.
    c. The patient is an alcoholic and needs a drink.
    d. The patient has developed physiologic dependence.

11. Match each pain characteristic with the type of pain it is most likely to be associated with.

Characteristic	Type of Pain
_____ Usually responds to commonly prescribed medical and nursing interventions	a. Acute pain
_____ May not be associated with an identified injury or event	b. Chronic pain
_____ Consists of discomfort lasting 1 to 2 months	
_____ Includes evidence of tissue damage	
_____ May not be reported	

12. A patient who has recently undergone surgery questions the use of narcotic analgesics and is concerned about becoming "hooked." Which response is most therapeutic?
    a. "You should avoid the use of narcotics after the first postoperative day to reduce the incidence of addiction."
    b. "Addiction is an unfortunate but common occurrence during the postoperative period."
    c. "Taking the ordered pain medicine every 6 hours will reduce the incidence of becoming addicted."
    d. "Becoming addicted to pain medication after short-term use is uncommon."
    e. "Do you have a history of alcohol or drug dependence?"

13. Which are associated with undertreatment of pain by health care providers? Select all that apply.

    _____ Concerns about the cost of medications prescribed

    _____ Inadequate information about the drugs ordered

    _____ Anxiety about potential patient injuries suffered while being medicated

    _____ Laziness of the health care provider

    _____ Concerns about fostering addiction

14. When administering nonopioid analgesics to a patient who has congestive heart failure, the nurse should perform what assessment to monitor for the presence of related adverse reactions?
    a. Intake and output
    b. Respiratory rate
    c. Temperature
    d. Cramping and diarrhea
    e. Superinfection

Exercise 2

Virtual Hospital Activity

20 minutes

- Sign in to work at Pacific View Regional Hospital for Period of Care 2. (*Note:* If you are already in the virtual hospital from a previous exercise, click on **Leave the Floor** and then on **Restart the Program** to get to the sign-in window.)
- From the Patient List, select Harry George (Room 401).
- Click on **Get Report** and read the shift report.

1. What are Harry George's medical diagnoses?

- Click on **Go to Nurses' Station** and then on **401** at the bottom of the screen.
- Click on and review the **Clinical Alerts**.

2. Harry George is reporting pain at a level of _____ on a _____-point scale.

3. The type of scale being used to assess Harry George's pain is known as a:
   a. visual analogue scale.
   b. numerical rating scale.
   c. verbal descriptor scale.
   d. linear pain continuum scale.

- Click on **Chart** and then on **401**.
- Click on and review the **Nursing Admission** and **History and Physical**.

- Click on **Return to Room 401**.
- Click on **MAR** and then on tab **401**.
- Review Harry George's ordered medications.

4. According to the nurse's entry on the MAR, Harry George may be remedicated for complaints of pain

   at _____.

5. How long after hydromorphone hydrochloride is administered to Harry George should interventions be performed to ensure maximum effectiveness of the drug? (*Hint:* Refer to the Drug Guide as necessary.)
   a. 10 minutes
   b. 15 to 30 minutes
   c. 30 to 60 minutes
   d. 2 hours
   e. 3 hours

6. If the administration route of the hydromorphone hydrochloride is changed to oral, what dosage of medication can be anticipated, assuming that Harry George's pain remains at the same level?
   a. 2.5 mg
   b. 7.5 mg
   c. 4 mg
   d. Cannot be determined.

7. Which medications are classified as opioid agonists? Select all that apply.

   _____ Codeine

   _____ Methadone

   _____ Buprenorphine (Buprenex)

   _____ Nalbuphine (Nubain)

   _____ Hydromorphone (Dilaudid)

   _____ Meperidine (Demerol)

8. Would an around-the-clock (ATC) or as-needed (PRN) method be most effective when administering analgesics to Harry George? Why?

9. Indicate whether each statement is true or false.

   a. _____ Hydromorphone has a ceiling effect on analgesia.

   b. _____ Harry George's physician has ordered his analgesics to be given every 3 hours PRN. The nurse may administer them ATC if the every-3-hours schedule is adhered to.

   c. _____ Nonopioids and opioids can be administered together.

   d. _____ The nurse cannot ask the unlicensed personnel to check on the level of pain being experienced by the patient.

10. Use the Sedation Scale to evaluate Harry George's current status. Which best identifies his status during this period of care?
    a. S
    b. 1
    c. 2
    d. 3
    e. 4

11. At what level on the sedation scale should a patient on opioids be?

12. When developing a plan of care for Harry George, a nurse knows that which nursing diagnosis is most appropriate and has the highest priority?
   a. Activity intolerance
   b. Ineffective role performance
   c. Ineffective coping
   d. Hopelessness
   e. Disturbed body image
   f. Acute pain

Exercise 3

Virtual Hospital Activity

20 minutes

- Sign in to work at Pacific View Regional Hospital for Period of Care 2. (*Note:* If you are already in the virtual hospital from a previous exercise, click on **Leave the Floor** and then on **Restart the Program** to get to the sign-in window.)
- From the Patient List, select Pablo Rodriguez (Room 405).
- Click on **Get Report** and read the shift report.
- Click on **Go to Nurses' Station** and then on **405** at the bottom of the screen.
- Click on **Take Vital Signs**.

   1. Presently, Pablo Rodriguez is reporting a pain level of _____ on a 10-point scale.

- Click on **Chart** and then on **405**.
- Click on and review the **Nursing Admission** and **History and Physical**.

   2. What are Pablo Rodriguez's medical diagnoses?

- Click on **Return to Room 405**.
- Click on **Patient Care** and then on **Physical Assessment**. Complete a head-to-toe assessment of Pablo Rodriguez by clicking on the body system categories (yellow buttons) and body system subcategories (green buttons).

3. Based on your assessment, which are sources of discomfort for Pablo Rodriguez? Select all that apply.

    _____   Condition of the oral cavity

    _____   Constipation

    _____   Ability to urinate

    _____   Breathing

    _____   Subcutaneous nodules

    _____   Lymph nodes in the neck

- Click on **EPR** and then on **Login**.
- Select **405** from the Patient drop-down menu and **Vital Signs** from the Category drop-down menu.
- Review the information concerning Pablo Rodriguez's pain during this hospitalization. Use the arrows at the bottom of the screen to view previous entries.

4. During this hospitalization, the range of reported pain levels for Pablo Rodriguez has been between

    _____ and _____.

5. Which characteristics are used to describe Pablo Rodriguez's pain on Wednesday? Select all that apply.

    _____   Aching

    _____   Burning

    _____   Chronic

    _____   Dull

    _____   Electric

    _____   Intermittent

    _____   Internal

    _____   Sharp

    _____   Shooting

- Click on **Exit EPR**.
- Click on **MAR** and then on tab **405**.
- Review Pablo Rodriguez's ordered medications.

6. Match each of Pablo Rodriguez's ordered medications with the corresponding classification.

Medication	Classification
_____ Morphine sulfate	a. Antiemetic; blocks serotonin
_____ Metoclopramide hydrochloride	b. Ammonia detoxicant
_____ Mineral oil	c. Schedule II narcotic analgesic
_____ Zolpidem	d. Stool softener
_____ Dexamethasone	e. Schedule IV hypnotic
_____ Senna	f. Antiemetic; reduces esophageal reflux
_____ Lactulose	g. Laxative
_____ Ondansetron	h. Corticosteroid

7. What is the rationale for ordering two analgesics to manage Pablo Rodriguez's pain?
   a. Providing the IV push medication will reduce his dependence on the patient-controlled analgesia (PCA) pump.
   b. Having multiple analgesic orders will allow him to choose which is preferred.
   c. This is a standard order.
   d. Having the two medications provides a means to manage breakthrough pain.

8. Opioids have been ordered to manage Pablo Rodriguez's pain. Which best describes the manner in which these medications work?
   a. Interfere with the relay of the pain signal across the synapse
   b. Inhibit prostaglandin synthesis
   c. Reduce serotonin availability to reduce pain occurrence
   d. Prevent and block the generation of the pain signals sent

9. Identify the potential side effects associated with opioid use. Select all that apply.

   _____ Diarrhea

   _____ Constipation

   _____ Drowsiness

   _____ Nausea

   _____ Hypertension

   _____ Bradycardia

   _____ Diaphoresis

10. What nonpharmacologic interventions can be used to manage Pablo Rodriguez's pain?

11. The MAR reports that Pablo Rodriguez has a continuous PCA pump with morphine sulfate PCA 1 mg/mL, 0.5 mg every 10 min/12 mg in 4-hour lockout. What is the maximum amount of morphine that may be delivered by the PCA pump in a 4-hour period?
    a. 10 mg
    b. 12 mg
    c. 6 mg
    d. 24 mg

12. How long after the administration of morphine sulfate via PCA pump should the patient's pain level be reevaluated?
    a. 5 minutes
    b. 15 minutes
    c. 30 minutes
    d. 45 minutes

13. When caring for Pablo Rodriguez, at what respiratory rate should morphine sulfate be held?
    a. 8 breaths per minute
    b. 10 breaths per minute
    c. 12 breaths per minute
    d. 14 breaths per minute

LESSON 6

Surgical Care

Reading Assignment: Surgical Care (Chapter 17)

Patient: Piya Jordan, Room 403

Objectives:

1. State the purpose of each type of surgery: diagnostic, exploratory, curative, palliative, and cosmetic.

2. List data to be included in the nursing assessment of the preoperative patient.

3. Assist in identifying the nursing diagnoses, goals, outcome criteria, and interventions during the preoperative phase of the surgical experience.

4. Outline a preoperative teaching plan.

5. List the responsibilities for each member of the surgical team.

6. Explain the nursing implications for each type of anesthesia.

7. Explain how the nurse can help prevent postoperative complications.

8. List data to be included in the nursing assessment of the postoperative patient.

9. Identify nursing diagnoses, goals, outcome criteria, and interventions for the postoperative patient.

10. Explain patient needs to be considered in discharge teaching.

Exercise 1

Writing Activity

45 minutes

1. Nurses who care for patients before, during, and after surgery are called _____ nurses.

2. Match each type of surgery with the corresponding definition.

Type of Surgery	Definition
_____ Diagnostic	a. Relieves symptoms or improves function without providing a solution to the basic problem
_____ Exploratory	b. Used to remove and study tissue to make a diagnosis
_____ Curative	c. Performed to correct defects that affect appearance
_____ Palliative	d. Used to diagnose and determine the extent of a disease process
_____ Cosmetic	e. Used to remove diseased tissue or to correct defects

3. Identify several variables that can affect surgical outcomes.

4. While preparing a patient for surgery, a nurse presents the surgical consent for the patient's signature. The patient reports he does not understand what the physician told him about the rationale for the procedure. Which response by the nurse is most appropriate?
   a. "This is just a formality. You can sign anyway."
   b. "Let me explain the procedure so that you can sign."
   c. "I will contact your physician so that you can ask for clarification."
   d. "You won't be able to get better without this surgery."

5. Which patients are able to provide informed consent for surgery? Select all that apply.

_____ A 101-year-old male

_____ A married 17-year-old female

_____ A 21-year-old female who has received preoperative medications

_____ A 17-year-old male

_____ A confused 34-year-old male

6. A patient is admitted to the clinical facility for an unexpected surgery. During the data collection, a nurse determines that the patient had toast and hot tea earlier in the day. How much preoperative fasting time is typically required before surgery after ingesting a meal of this type?
   a. 2 hours
   b. 4 hours
   c. 6 hours
   d. 8 hours
   e. Overnight

7. Match each type of anesthesia with the corresponding definition.

Anesthesia	Definition
_____ Local	a. Produced by inhalation or injection of anesthetic drugs into the bloodstream; causes a loss of all sensation and consciousness
_____ General	
_____ Regional	b. Injection of an agent into vessels; produces a lack of sensation over a specific body area
_____ Nerve block	
_____ Spinal	c. The temporary loss of feeling as a result of the inhibition of nerve endings in a specific part of the body
	d. Known as subarachnoid block; used for surgical procedures on the lower abdomen, perineum, and lower extremities
	e. The instillation of medication into or around the nerves to block the transmission of nerve impulses in a particular area or region

8. After administering spinal anesthesia, keeping the patient _____ may reduce the risk for developing a postprocedural headache.

9. The use of multiple drugs to manage a patient's anesthesia is referred to as _____

   _____.

10. During a surgical procedure, the physician reports that the patient is demonstrating signs consistent with malignant hyperthermia. Which manifestations are consistent with this phenomenon? Select all that apply.

_____ Increased systolic blood pressure

_____ Decreased diastolic blood pressure

_____ Tachycardia

_____ Muscle rigidity

_____ Cyanosis

_____ Increased body temperature

11. Which criteria must be met before discharging a patient who underwent conscious sedation? Select all that apply.

_____ Stable vital signs

_____ Intact motor function

_____ Tolerating ordered diet

_____ Ability to void

_____ Patent airway

12. _____ refers to the reopening of a surgical wound.

13. The protrusion of organs from an open wound is known as _____.

14. Match each type of wound drainage with the corresponding characteristic.

Drainage Type	**Characteristic**
_____ Serous	a. Pink, watery drainage consisting of plasma and red blood cells (RBCs)
_____ Sanguineous	b. Clear, watery plasma drainage
_____ Serosanguineous	c. A protein-rich drainage, which is the result of the liquefaction of necrotic tissue
_____ Purulent	d. Red drainage

15. A patient has a surgical wound in which a considerable amount of tissue was lost. The wound has healed with granulation tissue and epithelization. What type of healing has this wound demonstrated?
a. Primary intention
b. Secondary intention
c. Tertiary intention
d. Mixed intention

16. Indicate whether each statement is true or false.

    a. _____ A patient who had surgery 36 hours ago and currently has a temperature of 100.4° F is demonstrating the onset of an infection.

    b. _____ Older patients do not develop high fevers in the presence of an infection during the postoperative period.

17. If a surgical patient has a history of diabetes, which events associated with the condition may increase the risk for the development of complications? Select all that apply.

_____ Impaired tissue perfusion

_____ Increased RBC count

_____ Inhibition of leukocyte activity

_____ Reduced platelet count

_____ Slowed inflammatory response

Exercise 2

Virtual Hospital Activity

45 minutes

- Sign in to work at Pacific View Regional Hospital for Period of Care 1. (*Note:* If you are already in the virtual hospital from a previous exercise, click on **Leave the Floor** and then on **Restart the Program** to get to the sign-in window.)
- From the Patient List, select Piya Jordan (Room 403).
- Click on **Get Report** and read the shift report.
- Click on **Go to Nurses' Station**.
- Click on **Chart** and then on **403**.
- Click on and review the **Nursing Admission**.

1. Why has Piya Jordan come to the hospital?

2. How old is Piya Jordan?

3. Why do older patients have additional risks associated with surgery?

4. Piya Jordan's past medical history reflects disorders in which body systems? Select all that apply.

_____ Pulmonary

_____ Cardiovascular

_____ Renal

_____ Neurologic

_____ Metabolic

_____ Integumentary

_____ Gastrointestinal

_____ Musculoskeletal

• Click on and review the **Surgical Reports** and **Physician's Notes**.

5. What surgical procedure was performed on Piya Jordan?

6. Which surgical types describes the procedures performed on Piya Jordan? Select all that apply.

_____ Diagnostic

_____ Ablative

_____ Palliative

_____ Constructive

_____ Reconstructive

_____ Transplant

7. Piya Jordan had _____ anesthesia.

- Click on and review the **Laboratory Reports** and **Diagnostic Reports**.

8. Which laboratory tests were performed on Piya Jordan during the preoperative phase? Select all that apply.

_____ Complete blood count (CBC)

_____ Urinalysis

_____ Serum cholesterol levels

_____ Type and crossmatch

_____ Arterial blood gases (ABG)

_____ Electrolyte panel

9. Laboratory testing completed during Piya Jordan's preoperative period reflected some abnormal values. Which laboratory values were abnormal during the preoperative phase? Select all that apply.

_____ RBC count

_____ International normalized ration (INR)

_____ Potassium

_____ Sodium

_____ Hemoglobin

_____ Hematocrit

_____ Creatinine

_____ Prothrombin time (PT)

10. For which complication is Piya Jordan at risk because of her INR result?
    a. Urinary retention
    b. Pneumonia
    c. Paralytic ileus
    d. Hemorrhage

11. Which diagnostic tests were used to confirm the presence of an abdominal mass in Piya Jordan? Select all that apply.

_____ Chest x-ray

_____ Kidney-ureter-bladder x-ray (KUB)

_____ Infrared video pupillography (IVP)

_____ Colonoscopy

_____ Computed tomography (CT) scan of abdomen

12. _____ Piya Jordan has drug allergies that may influence the medications prescribed by the physician in both the preoperative and postoperative phases. (True/False)

• Click on **Surgical Reports** and **Expired MARs** and review the records.

13. Identify the sedative and antibiotic that Piya Jordan received preoperatively.

Name	**Dose**	**Route**

• Click on and review the **Physician's Orders**.

14. During the preoperative period, the physician ordered phytonadione 10 mg to be administered subcutaneously. Why was this medication ordered?

15. Identify the intervention used to prepare Piya Jordan's bowel for the operative procedure.
    a. Mineral oil enema
    b. Fleet enema
    c. Soap suds enema
    d. Oil retention enema
    e. No enema was administered because of the presence of the abdominal mass.

16. _____ Piya Jordan's home medications, digoxin and warfarin, can increase the effects of general anesthesia. (True/False)

17. During the surgical procedure, which responsibilities are included in the role of the circulating nurse? Select all that apply.

_____ Assessing the patient

_____ Setting up the surgical room

_____ Handling the instruments within the sterile field

_____ Providing assistance with patient positioning

_____ Monitoring for the use of aseptic technique

_____ Maintaining patient safety

18. Piya Jordan has an indwelling Foley catheter. Which best explains the rationale for the insertion of this catheter before surgery?
    a. The Foley catheter will allow for close monitoring of urinary output.
    b. Having a Foley catheter will allow the patient to rest instead of needing to walk to the bathroom or commode.
    c. The Foley catheter will reduce the occurrence of urinary tract infections (UTIs).
    d. The Foley catheter reduces the size of the bladder and reduces the chance for injury during the surgical procedure.

19. Piya Jordan has a Jackson-Pratt drain. Which statements about this device are correct? Select all that apply.

_____ It was placed in Piya Jordan's incision while she was in the Post-Anesthesia Care Unit (PACU).

_____ It will reduce fluid accumulation between surfaces of the wound.

_____ It is a small, pliable flat latex tube used to promote drainage.

_____ It is a closed drainage system.

_____ It is an open drainage system.

_____ It has a cartridge.

_____ It has a bulb.

- Click on **Return to Nurses' Station**.
- Click on **403** at the bottom of the screen.
- Review the Initial Observations.
- Click on **Patient Care** and then on **Physical Assessment**. Complete a systems assessment by clicking on the body system categories (yellow buttons) and body system subcategories (green buttons).

20. What should be included in the assessment of Piya Jordan's incision? Select all that apply.

_____ Approximation of the sutures

_____ Color of tissue surrounding the incision

_____ Presence of drainage from the incision

_____ Total number of sutures

_____ Odor of the incision

21. _____ During this period in the postoperative phase, Piya Jordan should use a heating pad on her incision to promote comfort. (True/False)

Intravenous Therapy

Reading Assignment: Intravenous Therapy (Chapter 18)

Patient: Patricia Newman, Room 406

Objectives:

1. List the indications for intravenous (IV) fluid therapy.

2. Describe the types of fluids used for IV fluid therapy.

3. Describe the types of venous access devices and other equipment used for IV therapy.

4. Explain the causes, signs and symptoms, and nursing implications of the complications of IV fluid or drug therapy.

5. Explain the nursing responsibilities when a patient is receiving IV therapy.

Exercise 1

Writing Activity

20 minutes

1. Fluids containing water and electrolytes are referred to as _____; fluids containing

   blood and blood products are called _____.

2. _____ *Tonicity* is the term used to measure the concentration of vitamins in an intravenous
   solution. (True/False)

3. A nurse is preparing an adult patient for an appendectomy. Which cannula size will be most appropriate
   to use?
   a. 14- to 16-gauge
   b. 18- to 20-gauge
   c. 22-gauge
   d. 24-gauge

4. A nurse is preparing to start an IV. Which tool may be used to assist in locating a vein?
   a. Transilluminator
   b. Veni-locator
   c. Transdermal lighting
   d. Intradermal lighting

5. Indicate whether each statement is true or false.

   a. _____ Presently, heparin is used to flush only central lines and not peripheral locks.

   b. _____ A round-corded tourniquet is most beneficial when starting an IV.

   c. _____ The use of normal saline injections at the IV site to provide anesthesia is a widely used
   practice.

6. When selecting a site for IV insertion, the nurse should begin with the most _____

   site and move _____ as needed.

7. When preparing to start an IV, which are contradictions to the use of an extremity? Select all that apply.

_____ It is the patient's dominant hand.

_____ There is impaired circulation in the extremity.

_____ There is impaired lymphatic drainage in the extremity.

_____ The patient has an arteriovenous (AV) graft in the extremity.

_____ The patient has a history of a mastectomy on the same side as the extremity.

_____ Blood work was obtained from the extremity within the last 4 hours.

8. A patient asks a nurse whether antibiotic ointment should be used at the site of her IV insertion. Which is the best response to the patient's question?
   a. "There is no risk for developing an infection at the insertion site."
   b. "The cleaning of the site adequately sterilized it."
   c. "There is some controversy concerning that practice. I will need to consult with your physician."
   d. "I will apply antibiotic ointment during my next assessment."

9. When monitoring the flow rate for an IV infusion, a nurse must recognize factors that affect the infusion rate. Which statements concerning IV infusions are correct? Select all that apply.

_____ Lowering the IV bag will increase the flow rate.

_____ A full infusion bag will infuse more rapidly.

_____ Viscous fluids will flow more rapidly.

_____ Venting rigid containers is necessary to ensure flow.

_____ Larger cannulas will promote a more rapid rate of infusion.

10. Permission for a licensed practical nurse (LPN) to administer IV push medications is determined by the

_____ _____ _____ of the individual state in which the LPN is practicing.

11. Identify at least three indications for the administration of IV fluids.

12. The patient has had a central line placed by the surgeon. Which statement by the patient indicates an understanding of the line and related care?
   a. "I will have to have the location of my line checked by the radiologist."
   b. An infusion of normal saline will be administered before medications to ensure the line is in the correct vessel."
   c. "I will need to have this line changed every 3 to 4 months."
   d. "A magnet can be used to determine placement of the line."

Exercise 2

Virtual Hospital Activity

45 minutes

- Sign in to work at Pacific View Regional Hospital for Period of Care 2. (*Note:* If you are already in the virtual hospital from a previous exercise, click on **Leave the Floor** and then on **Restart the Program** to get to the sign-in window.)
- From the Patient List, select Patricia Newman (Room 406).
- Click on **Get Report** and read the shift report.
- Click on **Go to Nurses' Station**.
- Click on **Chart** and then on **406**.
- Click on and review the **Nursing Admission** and **Laboratory Reports**.

1. Why was Patricia Newman admitted to the hospital?

2. Patricia Newman has a serum potassium level of _____ mEq/L.

3. The normal range for serum potassium levels is:
    a. 3.0-4.5 mEq/L.
    b. 3.5-5.1 mEq/L.
    c. 3.5-5.5 mEq/L.
    d. 4.0-6.5 mEq/L.

- Click on and review the **Physician's Notes** and **Physician's Orders**.

4. What IV fluids have been ordered by the physician?

5. Which are roles of potassium in the body? Select all that apply.

_____ Protein synthesis

_____ Regulation of acid-base balance

_____ Maintenance of fluid osmolarity and volume within the cell

_____ Transmission of nerve impulses

_____ Metabolism of carbohydrates

_____ Synthesis and breakdown of glycogen

6. The physician has ordered the IV solution to infuse at _____ mL/hour.

7. How many mL of fluids will Patricia Newman receive in a 24-hour period?

8. How many calories will be provided to Patricia Newman from a liter of IV fluids?
   a. 100
   b. 150
   c. 170
   d. 190
   e. 200
   f. 340

9. What classification can best be used to describe Patricia Newman's prescribed IV fluids?
   a. Isotonic
   b. Hypotonic
   c. Hypertonic

10. Based on the standards of the Intravenous Nurses Society, how frequently should Patricia Newman's IV tubing be changed?
   a. Every 24 hours
   b. Every 48 to 72 hours
   c. Weekly
   d. Only when problems arise

• Click on **Return to Nurses' Station** and then on **406** at the bottom of the screen.
• Click on **Check Armband**.
• Review the Initial Observations.
• Click on **Patient Care** and then on **Physical Assessment**. Complete an assessment of the IV site by clicking on the body system categories (yellow buttons) and body system subcategories (green buttons).

11. Patricia Newman is _____ years of age.

12. Older patients may require special observations related to the administration of intravenous fluids. Identify some common issues regarding IV administration unique to the older adult population.

13. When assessing Patricia Newman's IV site, the nurse knows that which manifestations are consistent with infiltration? Select all that apply.

_____ Warmth at IV site

_____ Coolness at IV site

_____ Fluid leakage around site of cannula insertion

_____ Paleness in the skin surrounding site of insertion

_____ Edema surrounding site of insertion

14. _____ Patricia Newman's IV site demonstrates symptoms consistent with early-onset infiltration. (True/False)

15. If an IV site infiltrates, what care should be provided to the affected extremity?
    a. Elevate the extremity
    b. Position the extremity lower than the level of the heart
    c. Wrap the extremity in an ace wrap to prevent further absorption of fluids into the surrounding tissues
    d. Apply ice pack treatments to reduce neurologic damage to the extremity

16. What term would best be used to describe Patricia Newman's IV?
    a. Peripheral
    b. Midline
    c. Peripheral venous catheterization (PVC)
    d. Peripherally inserted central catheter (PICC)
    e. Central venous catheter (CVC)

17. Review Patricia Newman's condition. What are the underlying rationales for her IV therapy?

- Click on **MAR** and then on tab **406** and review Patricia Newman's scheduled medications.

18. Identify the medication that will be administered via IV.

19. The preceding medication will be administered _____.

20. The total volume that will be infused with the IV medication will be _____ mL.

21. The IV medication is premixed in a _____ solution.

22. Before administering cefotetan to Patricia Newman, a nurse must assess for which item?
    a. Sensitivity to penicillin
    b. Sensitivity to acetylsalicylic acid (ASA)
    c. Corticosteroid use
    d. History of phlebitis

Loss, Death, and End-of-Life Care

Reading Assignment: Loss, Death, and End-of-Life Care (Chapter 24)

Patient: Pablo Rodriguez, Room 405

Objectives:

1. Understand the beliefs and practices related to death and dying.

2. Describe the responses of patients and their families to terminal illness and death.

3. Identify and discuss nursing interventions for meeting the needs of terminally ill, dying patients and their significant others.

4. Discuss directives related to caring for the dying patient, including advance directives, do-not-resuscitate decisions, brain death, organ donation, and pronouncement of death.

Exercise 1

Writing Activity

20 minutes

1. Grief that is delayed or exaggerated may be identified as _____.

2. Match each age group with its associated beliefs and attitudes about death.

Age Group	**Belief/Attitude**
_____ Preschoolers	a. Death is seen as unavoidable.
_____ School-age children	b. Religious beliefs have the greatest influence on beliefs concerning death.
_____ Preadolescents	c. Death can be reversed.
_____ Adolescents	d. Fear of experiencing a prolonged death may be present.
_____ Young adults	e. Death anxiety may be experienced.
_____ Middle adults	f. Death is the result of a violent act.
_____ Older adults	g. Attitudes concerning death are based on those of adults in their network.

3. A woman is displaying anger about the impending death of her terminally ill husband. According to Martocchio's grief cluster of yearning and protest, toward whom may this anger be focused? Select all that apply.

_____ Her husband

_____ God

_____ The nursing staff

_____ Herself

_____ The physician

4. Listed below are the stages of death and dying according to Elisabeth Kübler-Ross. Match the two columns to place each stage in its order of occurrence.

Stage	Order of Occurrence
_____ Acceptance	a. Stage 1
_____ Bargaining	b. Stage 2
_____ Denial	c. Stage 3
_____ Depression	d. Stage 4
_____ Anger	e. Stage 5

5. While providing assistance to the spouse of a patient diagnosed with a terminal illness, a nurse notes that the spouse is having difficulty making decisions and has a lack of interest in the future. Which of the grief clusters, as defined by Martocchio, is being manifested?
   a. Shock and disbelief
   b. Yearning and protest
   c. Anguish, disorganization, and despair
   d. Identification in bereavement
   e. Reorganization and restitution

6. A nurse is providing emotional support to the parents of a young car crash victim who is not expected to live. Which physical manifestations and/or emotions can the nurse anticipate the parents to experience? Select all that apply.

   _____ Shortness of breath

   _____ An overwhelming sense of strength to manage the situation

   _____ Tightness in the chest

   _____ Feelings of suffocation

   _____ Feelings of emptiness

7. While working with the family of a patient who is nearing death, a nurse should use which statements to facilitate the interaction? Select all that apply.

   _____ "You are being so strong."

   _____ "I know how you feel."

   _____ "I will keep you in my thoughts."

   _____ "Time will make it easier."

   _____ "You must get on with your life."

8. Which may be viewed as risk factors for experiencing a maladaptive grief process? Select all that apply.

   _____ Dependent relationships

   _____ A lengthy terminal illness

   _____ History of alcohol abuse

   _____ Current history of substance abuse

   _____ Cumulative grief over multiple unresolved losses

9. Written statements that identify a patient's wishes concerning medical care are known as

   _____ _____.

10. What is the Patient Self-Determination Act?

11. A recent widow is working through Rando's phases of mourning. What activities are consistent with a positive movement through the stage of confrontation?
    a. She begins to discuss the feelings of becoming a widow with her friends and family.
    b. She joins a support group for new widows.
    c. She contacts a local community college about enrolling in courses.
    d. She donates clothing of the deceased to a local charity.

12. The nurse is caring for a patient who is nearing death. The patient's spouse has indicated that the patient and family are Orthodox Jews who will be following traditional customs. Which activities may be included in this patient's end-of-life and death care? Select all that apply.

   _____ The patient will be left alone for a short period after death for spiritual "settling."

   _____ The body will be washed by an older female relative.

   _____ Burial must occur within 24 hours.

   _____ The dying patient is not to be left alone.

   _____ The body must not be touched for up to 30 minutes after death.

13. When caring for the recently deceased what actions by the nurse are appropriate? Select all that apply.

_____ Place the deceased hands at their sides.

_____ Rest the head and shoulders on a large fluffy pillow.

_____ Insert the patient's dentures.

_____ Gently hold the eyelids closed to aid them in staying closed.

_____ Remove any connected IV tubing

Exercise 2

Virtual Hospital Activity

30 minutes

- Sign in to work at Pacific View Regional Hospital for Period of Care 1. (*Note:* If you are already in the virtual hospital from a previous exercise, click on **Leave the Floor** and then on **Restart the Program** to get to the sign-in window.)
- From the Patient List, select Pablo Rodriguez (Room 405).
- Click on **Get Report** and read the shift report.
- Click on **Go to Nurses' Station**.
- Click on **Chart** and then **405**.
- Click on and review the **History and Physical**.

1. Why has Pablo Rodriguez been admitted to the hospital?

2. What are Pablo Rodriguez's medical diagnoses?

3. Which term best describes Pablo Rodriguez's mental state at the time of admission?
   a. Denial
   b. Resolved
   c. Depressed
   d. Anxious
   e. Nervous
   f. Angry

- Click on and review the **Nursing Admission**.

4. Which statement best describes the status of Pablo Rodriguez's advance directive?
   a. Pablo Rodriguez has executed an advance directive.
   b. Pablo Rodriguez has provided the hospital with a copy of his advance directive.
   c. Pablo Rodriguez has reported the existence of an advance directive and his intent to provide a copy to the hospital.
   d. Pablo Rodriguez has not executed an advance directive.
   e. Pablo Rodriguez has been provided written information about his rights regarding advance directives.

5. As Pablo Rodriguez begins to make decisions about his health care and end-of-life care, what will be needed to implement these decisions?
   a. Pablo Rodriguez will need to meet with his attorney to draft his living will.
   b. A notary will need to authenticate signatures on the living will document.
   c. Once Pablo Rodriguez physician agrees with his requested plan of care, it can be authorized.
   d. Pablo Rodriguez may provide verbal instructions to his physician with witnesses about his health care decisions.

6. In the event that a party is required to "step forward" to assist with decision making regarding Pablo Rodriguez's medical care, who will take on this role?
   a. Pablo Rodriguez's spouse
   b. The hospital attorney
   c. Pablo Rodriguez's physician
   d. The hospital's ethics committee
   e. Pablo Rodriguez's daughter
   f. Pablo Rodriguez's son

7. If religious council or sacraments are requested by Pablo Rodriguez or his family, which would most likely be consulted?
   a. A protestant minister
   b. A priest
   c. A rabbi
   d. A shaman

- Click on **Return to Nurses' Station** and then on **405** at the bottom of the screen.
- Review the Initial Observations.
- Click on **Patient Care** and then on **Nurse-Client Interactions**.
- Select and view the video titled **0730: Symptom Management**. (*Note:* Check the virtual clock to see whether enough time has elapsed. You can use the fast-forward feature to advance the time by 2-minute intervals if the video is not yet available. Then click again on **Patient Care** and **Nurse-Client Interactions** to refresh the screen.)

8. Which adjective best describes Pablo Rodriguez's ability to share his concerns?
   a. Hesitant
   b. Eager
   c. Open
   d. Nervous

9. Discuss Pablo Rodriguez's beliefs about how he became ill.

10. What value would sharing his feelings have for Pablo Rodriguez?
   a. An opportune time to bond with his loved ones
   b. A sign of weakness
   c. A waste of time
   d. A key step in preparing for his death

• Click on **Kardex** and then on tab **405**.

11. How long has Pablo Rodriguez been ill?

12. Pablo Rodriguez's code status is identified as:
   a. full code.
   b. partial code—medications only.
   c. partial code—cardiopulmonary resuscitation (CPR) only.
   d. Do not resuscitate (DNR).

13. If the 5 Wishes document were used for Pablo Rodriguez, what items would it contain?

The Patient with Cancer

Reading Assignment: The Patient with Cancer (Chapter 25)

Patient: Pablo Rodriguez, Room 405

Objectives:

1. Explain the differences between benign and malignant tumors.

2. List the most common sites of cancer in men and women.

3. Describe measures to reduce the risk for cancer.

4. List nursing responsibilities for the care of patients having diagnostic tests to detect possible cancer.

5. Explain the nursing care of patients undergoing various types of cancer therapy: surgery, radiation, chemotherapy, and biotherapy.

Exercise 1

Writing Activity

45 minutes

1. Specific characteristics are used to differentiate benign cells from malignant cells. Match each characteristic to the cellular category with which it is most closely associated.

Characteristic	**Cellular Category**
_____ A distinct recognizable appearance	a. Benign
_____ Ability to perform a specific function	b. Malignant
_____ The presence of multiple nuclei	
_____ Nuclei that are large in size	
_____ Nuclei that are small in size	
_____ Cell division inhibited by inadequate space and insufficient nutrients	
_____ Cells not readily recognized by other cells	
_____ Cells continue to divide despite space constraints	

2. _____ _____ is the term used to describe the movement of cancer cells into adjoining tissue.

3. List factors that may promote the transformation of normal cells into malignant cells.

4. Which foods have been shown to reduce the risk for developing cancer? Select all that apply.

    _____ Broccoli

    _____ Lettuce

    _____ Bananas

    _____ Carrots

    _____ Grapefruit

    _____ Tomatoes

5. A 40-year-old man has been diagnosed with esophageal cancer. Which factor is most likely to be in his personal history?
    a. Obesity
    b. A diet low in fiber
    c. A diet high in saturated fats
    d. A diet high in nitrates

6. A 21-year-old woman who is sexually active who has had negative Pap smears for the last 4 years and has no other risk factors asks how frequently she should have a Pap smear. Based on your knowledge, which time frame should the nurse give this patient?
    a. Annually
    b. Every 2 years
    c. Every 3 years
    d. Every 6 months

7. A patient asks at what age she should have her first mammogram. A review of the patient's history elicits no significant risk factors. What is the recommended age for the patient's initial mammogram?
    a. 25 years of age
    b. 30 years of age
    c. 40 years of age
    d. 45 years of age

8. When providing care to an African-American male, the nurse should be aware that which cancers are most prevalent in this population? Select all that apply.

   _____ Oral

   _____ Prostate

   _____ Breast

   _____ Colon

   _____ Integumentary

   _____ Rectal

   _____ Lung

9. Match each diagnostic test with the corresponding description.

   Diagnostic Test

   _____ Computed tomography (CT)

   _____ Radionuclide scans

   _____ Ultrasound testing

   _____ Magnetic resonance imaging (MRI)

   Description

   a. Noninvasive, high-frequency sound waves are used to examine external body structures.

   b. A computer processes radio-frequency energy waves to assess spinal lesions, as well as cardiovasculat and soft tissue abnormalities.

   c. Radiographs and computed scanning are used to provide images of structures at differing angles.

   d. A substance is injected; the uptake is evaluated to identify areas of concern.

10. _____ therapy is used when a patient who has had surgery or radiotherapy is free of signs of disease but has a high risk for recurrence of the disease.

11. Before radiation therapy, the physician marks the skin of the patient. Which instructions should be provided to the patient concerning these markings?
    a. "You may wash these marks with soap and water after this treatment."
    b. "Use a mild solution of rubbing alcohol and water to remove these marks."
    c. "Do not remove these marks."
    d. "Use lotion to soften the skin around these marks if needed."

12. A patient undergoing treatment for cancer has experienced alopecia. Which should be included in information to the patient concerning this occurrence? Select all that apply.

    _____ The hair color may be different after regrowth.

    _____ The texture of new hair growth will mimic that of the original hair.

    _____ The alopecia is temporary.

    _____ Medications may assist in limiting the amount of hair lost.

    _____ Alopecia may be partial or total.

13. The complete blood cell profile of a patient diagnosed with cancer shows a reduction in the number of circulating platelets. Which term is used to describe this condition?
    a. Leukopenia
    b. Thrombocytopenia
    c. Anemia
    d. Neutropenia

14. A patient undergoing radiation treatment reports that he is perspiring and asks what can be done to manage this problem. Which response should be included in information provided to the patient?
    a. "You may use deodorant but not antiperspirant."
    b. "The use of antiperspirants is allowed."
    c. "You may use corn starch to absorb the moisture."
    d. "There is nothing that can be done to manage this problem."

15. _____ _____ is a complex metabolic problem characterized by weight loss, anemia, and abnormalities in fat, protein, and carbohydrate metabolism.

16. Nontraditional therapies combined with conventional therapies are known as _____.

    Therapies used in lieu of traditional therapies are termed _____.

17. What are the three most common types of cancer found in men?

18. Match the type of malignant tumor with the corresponding tissue of origin.

Malignant Tumor Type	Tissue of Origin
_____ Melanoma	a. Skin, glands, linings of digestive, urinary, and respiratory tracts
_____ Sarcoma	b. Bone, muscle, other connective tissue
_____ Carcinoma	c. Pigment cells in the skin
_____ Leukemia and lymphomas	d. Blood forming tissues

Exercise 2

Virtual Hospital Activity

45 minutes

- Sign in to work at Pacific View Regional Hospital for Period of Care 2. (*Note:* If you are already in the virtual hospital from a previous exercise, click on **Leave the Floor** and then on **Restart the Program** to get to the sign-in window.)
- From the Patient List, select Pablo Rodriguez (Room 405).
- Click on **Get Report** and read the shift report.
- Click on **Go to Nurses' Station** and then on **405** at the bottom of the screen.
- Click on and review the **Clinical Alerts**.
- Click on **Chart** and then on **405**.
- Click on and review the **Nursing Admission** and **History and Physical**.

1. What are Pablo Rodriguez's medical diagnoses?

2. What were Pablo Rodriguez's chief complaints at the time of admission?

- Click on and review the **Physician's Orders**.

3. Beginning in the Emergency Department, what interventions were implemented to address the Pablo Rodriguez's chief complaints?

- Click again on **Nursing Admission**.

4. How does Pablo Rodriguez report his prognosis?

5. Given Pablo Rodriguez's advanced cancer and his beliefs that his death is near, what actions by additional referrals may be indicated to assist him and his family?

6. _____ Pablo Rodriguez has a positive family history of cancer. (True/False)

7. Based on information reported in the Nursing Admission, what physiologic changes have taken place as a result of the cancer?

8. Which methods of treatment does Pablo Rodriguez report using to manage his cancer? Select all that apply.

_____ Surgery

_____ Radiation

_____ Chemotherapy

_____ Alternative therapies

_____ Complementary therapies

9. _____ is a means of treating cancer that can be used to reduce or slow the growth of metastatic cells.

10. Which best describe the modes of action and uses for radiation therapy? Select all that apply.

_____ May be administered internally

_____ May be administered externally

_____ Used exclusively for palliative care

_____ Used to treat cancer that cannot be surgically removed

_____ Used to manage cancer that has spread to local lymph nodes

• Click on and review the **Physician's Orders** and **Physician's Notes**.

11. The physician has ordered a low-fat, bland diet. Which items will Pablo Rodriguez be allowed to include in this diet? Select all that apply.

_____ Organ meats

_____ Toast

_____ Baked chicken

_____ Broth

_____ Milk shakes

_____ Tacos

12. Discuss the implications of this diet on Pablo Rodriguez's preferred foods.

• Click on and review the **Laboratory Reports**.

13. Pablo Rodriguez's hemoglobin level is reduced. What factors may be associated with the presence of anemia? Select all that apply.

_____ Dehydration

_____ A low red blood cell (RBC) count

_____ A lack of hemoglobin in the erythrocytes

_____ Fluid retention

_____ Recent infection

14. Indicate whether each statement is true or false.

a. _____ Pablo Rodriguez's platelet levels are abnormal.

b. _____ Pablo Rodriguez's white blood cell (WBC) count is reduced, reflecting immunosuppression.

15. Which complaint voiced by Pablo Rodriguez can be attributed directly to the results reflected in the complete blood count (CBC)?
a. Nausea
b. Vomiting
c. Constipation
d. Fatigue

16. Pablo Rodriguez had an electrolyte panel drawn. Which of his electrolyte values are abnormal? Select all that apply.

_____ Sodium

_____ Potassium

_____ Chloride

_____ Calcium

_____ Phosphorus

_____ Magnesium

- Click on **Return to Room 405**.
- Click on **Patient Care** and then on **Physical Assessment**. Complete a head-to-toe assessment of Pablo Rodriguez by clicking on the body system categories (yellow buttons) and body system subcategories (green buttons).

17. At the time of his admission, Pablo Rodriguez reported being unable to tolerate oral intake. What assessment findings support this report?

- Click on **Chart** and then on **405**.
- Click on and review the **Physician's Orders**.

18. What medications were ordered to manage Pablo Rodriguez's nausea?

19. The medications listed have been prescribed for Pablo Rodriguez. Match each drug with its correct classification/use.

Medication	Classification/Use
_____ Morphine sulfate	a. Laxative
_____ Metoclopramide hydrochloride	b. Narcotic analgesic
_____ Dexamethasone	c. Schedule IV hypnotic
_____ Senna	d. Corticosteroid, systemic
_____ Lactulose	e. Laxative, ammonia detoxicant
_____ Neutra-Phos	f. Antiemetic
_____ Ondansetron	g. Laxative; exerts osmotic effect in small intestine
_____ Zolpidem	h. Antiemetic

20. The physician prescribed ondansetron hydrochloride for Pablo Rodriguez. Which side effects associated with this medication may further complicate problems the patient is currently having? Select all that apply.

_____ Fatigue

_____ Excitability

_____ Diarrhea

_____ Urinary retention

_____ Constipation

_____ Blurred vision

21. In addition to opioids, what mediations may be used in the management of cancer pain?

Acute and Chronic Respiratory Disorders

Reading Assignment: Acute Disorders of the Lower Respiratory Tract (Chapter 31)
Chronic Disorders of the Lower Respiratory Tract (Chapter 32)

Patients: Jacquline Catanazaro, Room 402
Patricia Newman, Room 406

Objectives:

1. Identify data to be collected in the nursing assessment of a patient with a respiratory disorder.

2. Identify the nursing implications of age-related changes in the respiratory system.

3. Describe diagnostic tests or procedures for respiratory disorders and nursing interventions.

4. Explain nursing care of patients receiving therapeutic treatments for respiratory disorders.

5. Discuss the pathophysiology, signs and symptoms, complications, diagnostic measures, and medical treatment for identified respiratory disorders.

Exercise 1

Writing Activity

45 minutes

1. The normal respiratory rate in the adult is between _____ and _____ breaths per minute.

2. Match each respiratory disorder with the corresponding description.

Respiratory Disorder	**Description**
_____ Atelectasis	a. Inflammation of the lung with consolidation and exudation
_____ Pleural effusion	b. Accumulation of fluid in the space between the visceral visceral pleura and parietal pleura of the thorax
_____ Hemothorax	c. A collapsed or airless state of the lung or portion of a lung
_____ Pneumothorax	
_____ Pneumonia	d. An infectious, inflammatory, reportable disease that is chronic and commonly affects the lungs, although it may occur in other areas of the body
_____ Asthma	e. An inflammatory response that constricts the bronchi, causing edema and increased sputum
_____ Emphysema	
_____ Tuberculosis	f. Bleeding into the pleural space secondary to chest trauma
	g. Pathologic accumulation of air in tissues or organs
	h. Air from the lung leaking into the pleural space or chest

3. During shift report, an outgoing nurse advises you that a patient is demonstrating Kussmaul's respirations. Based on your knowledge, you recognize that the patient's respiratory patterns likely have which characteristics? Select all that apply.

_____ A regular pattern

_____ Periods of apnea

_____ Deep, uneven respirations

_____ A respiratory rate greater than 20 breaths/minute

_____ Tachypnea

4. After administration of an analgesic, which type of respiratory pattern would you anticipate the patient to exhibit?
   a. Biot's
   b. Kussmaul's
   c. Cheyne-Stokes
   d. Tachypnea
   e. Bradypnea

5. Describe changes associated with aging that may increase the potential for complications in the older adult patient.

6. While caring for a patient demonstrating a productive cough, a nurse must record the

   characteristics of the sputum. These characteristics include _____,

   _____, _____, and _____.

7. When performing a respiratory assessment, a nurse must remember that the presence of flaring nostrils

   is a manifestation associated with _____ _____.

8. Chest physiotherapy consists of _____, _____, and

   _____ drainage.

9. _____ Chest physiotherapy can be performed only by a respiratory therapist. (True/False)

10. Match each respiratory sound with the corresponding description.

Sound	Description
_____ Rhonchus	a. A high-pitched sound caused by air passing through narrowed passages
_____ Crackle	
_____ Coarse crackle	b. An abnormal sound similar to that made by rubbing pieces of hair between the finger
_____ Wheeze	c. A sound similar to Velcro pulling apart
_____ Pleural friction rub	d. A dry, rattling sound
	e. A grating, scratchy sound similar to a creaking shoe

11. A nurse is preparing to suction a patient. Which steps/concepts should be included in the process? Select all that apply.

_____ Use clean technique.

_____ Administer oxygen before initiating the intervention.

_____ Administer oxygen after completing the intervention.

_____ Apply suction as the catheter is withdrawn from the airway.

_____ Limit each suction attempt to 10 seconds.

_____ Complete the full cycle of suctioning before allowing the patient to rest.

_____ Document the patient's toleration of the procedure.

12. The physician has ordered percussion for a patient. For which conditions would this plan be contraindicated? Select all that apply.

_____ Pulmonary embolus

_____ Asthma

_____ Pneumonia

_____ Lung cancer

_____ Bronchospasm

13. Match each diagnostic test with the corresponding description.

Diagnostic Test

_____ Chest radiography

_____ Fluoroscopy

_____ Pulmonary function

_____ Thoracentesis

_____ Fiberoptic bronchoscopy

_____ Magnetic resonance imaging (MRI)

Description

a. Radiograph of the chest taken to observe deep structures in motion

b. Removal of pleural fluid for examination

c. Produces images of multiple body planes without radiation; used to detect abnormalities, lesions, and tumors

d. Used to screen and diagnose some respiratory disorders

e. Used to visualize abnormalities, take biopsy samples of lesions, or remove foreign bodies

f. Evaluates gas exchanges, pulmonary blood flow, and acid-base balance

14. A nurse is providing care to a patient who has had a bronchoscopy. Which position is most therapeutic?
   a. High Fowler
   b. Semi-Fowler
   c. Supine
   d. Prone

15. A patient is demonstrating hypoventilation. Which partial pressure of carbon dioxide ($PaCO_2$) results can be anticipated?
   a. Less than 31 mm Hg
   b. 32 to 40 mm Hg
   c. 40 mm Hg
   d. 47 mm Hg

16. Regarding the use of intermittent positive-pressure breathing (IPPB) treatments, which statements are correct? Select all that apply.

   _____ IPPB is used to achieve maximal lung expansion.

   _____ IPPB delivers humidified gas with negative pressure.

   _____ IPPB forces air into the lungs with inhalation.

   _____ IPPB allows passive exhalation.

   _____ IPPB results in a nonproductive cough.

Exercise 2

Virtual Hospital Activity

45 minutes

- Sign in to work at Pacific View Regional Hospital for Period of Care 1. (*Note:* If you are already in the virtual hospital from a previous exercise, click on **Leave the Floor** and then on **Restart the Program** to get to the sign-in window.)
- From the Patient List, select Jacquline Catanazaro (Room 402).
- Click on **Get Report** and read the shift report.
- Click on **Go to Nurses' Station**.
- Click on **Chart** and then on **402**.
- Click on and review the **Nursing Admission** and **History and Physical**.

1. What are Jacquline Catanazaro's medical diagnoses?

2. Which risk factors for the development of respiratory illness are noted in Jacquline Catanazaro's history? Select all that apply.

_____ Age

_____ History of travel

_____ Occupational exposures

_____ Smoking

_____ Family history

_____ Inactivity

3. _____ Jacquline Catanazaro's racial background is typical of most asthma sufferers. (True/False)

4. When managing the care of a patient suspected of having asthma, which tests may be ordered to confirm a diagnosis? Select all that apply.

_____ Complete blood count (CBC)

_____ Serum electrolyte levels

_____ Arterial blood gas (ABG)

_____ Pulmonary function tests

_____ Sputum cultures

• Click on and review the **Diagnostic Reports** and **Laboratory Reports**.

5. Jacquline Catanazaro had ABGs drawn on Tuesday at 0730. Which documented results were abnormal? Select all that apply.

_____ Partial pressure of oxygen (PaO_2)

_____ Oxygen (O_2) saturation

_____ $PaCO_2$

_____ Hydrogen ion concentration (pH)

• Click on **Return to Nurses' Station** and then on **402** at the bottom of the screen.
• Review the Initial Observations.
• Click on and review the **Clinical Alerts**.
• Click on **Take Vital Signs** and review the findings.

6. What is Jacquline Catanazaro's pulse oximeter reading?

7. What does the pulse oximeter reading reflect?
   a. Blood's hematocrit (Hct) level
   b. O_2 saturation of hemoglobin (Hgb) in the blood
   c. Body's level of $PaCO_2$
   d. Body's acid-base balance

8. When obtaining pulse oximeter readings on Jacquline Catanazaro, the nurse may use which sites? Select all that apply.

_____ Ear lobe

_____ Bridge of nose

_____ Tip of the nose

_____ Finger

_____ Toe

9. A saturation reading of _____% is the critical value for oxygenation to support life.

10. What factors may affect pulse oximeter readings? Select all that apply.

_____ Hypertension

_____ Vasodilation

_____ Hyperthermia

_____ Dark-colored nail polish

_____ Finger movement

• Click on **Patient Care** and then on **Physical Assessment**. Complete a systems assessment by clicking on the body system categories (yellow buttons) and body system subcategories (green buttons).

11. Identify any abnormalities found during Jacquline Catanazaro's respiratory assessment.

12. Jacquline Catanazaro has "crackles" noted in her lung assessment. What sound is characteristic to this type of phenomena?
   a. Continuous sonorous sounds
   b. High-pitched musical tones
   c. Low-pitched whistling sounds
   d. Bubbling sounds

13. What term that may be used interchangeably with "crackles"?
   a. Rhonchi
   b. Wheezes
   c. Friction
   d. Alveolar popping

14. The respiratory assessment reflects the presence of wheezes. What best describes the underlying cause of the wheezing sound?
   a. Pulmonary hypoventilation
   b. Mucus in the bronchioles
   c. Inflammation of the pleura
   d. Bronchoconstriction
   e. Fluid overload

15. Jacquline Catanazaro is demonstrating an increased respiratory rate. What factors can result in an increase in respiratory rate? Select all that apply.

_____ Exercise

_____ Fever

_____ Alkalosis

_____ Hypoxemia

_____ Hypercapnia

16. Jacquline Catanazaro's skin is noted as being moist and clammy. What significance does this have in relation to her respiratory status?

17. Jacquline Catanazaro's condition is consistent with the late phase of an asthmatic attack. What factors are characteristic of this phase? Select all that apply.

_____ Airway inflammation is reduced.

_____ Airway inflammation is pronounced.

_____ RBCs have infiltrated swollen tissues.

_____ This phase typically lasts only a few hours.

_____ The patient is at a heightened risk for an acute asthmatic attack.

18. Jacquline Catanazaro is demonstrating extreme agitation. What is the impact of these behaviors on her condition?

- Click on **Patient Care** and then on **Nurse-Client Interactions**.
- Select and view the video titled **0730: Intervention—Airway**. (*Note:* Check the virtual clock to see whether enough time has elapsed. You can use the fast-forward feature to advance the time by 2-minute intervals if the video is not yet available. Then click again on **Patient Care** and **Nurse-Client Interactions** to refresh the screen.)

19. Jacquline Catanazaro is experiencing an acute asthma attack. What has been planned to manage the onset?

- Click on **Chart** and then on **402**.
- Click on the **Physician's Orders** tab and note the admission orders for Monday at 1600.

20. What medications have been ordered to manage Jacquline Catanazaro's respiratory condition? For each medication, include the dose and route of administration ordered.

- Click **Return to Room 402** and then click on the **Drug** icon.
- Review the information for the drugs that have been prescribed for Jacquline Catanazaro.

21. For each medication identified in the previous question, list the mode of action.

22. When providing patient education concerning the use of beclomethasone, the nurse should tell the patient that which side effects may occur?
    a. Throat irritation
    b. Productive cough
    c. Increased pulmonary secretions
    d. Skin rash
    e. Activity intolerance

23. When preparing Jacquline Catanazaro for discharge to home, which concepts should be included in the education provided? Select all that apply.

    _____   Understand the prescribed drug therapy.

    _____   Limit water intake to reduce pulmonary edema.

    _____   Promptly report infections to physicians.

    _____   If symptoms occur during exercise, suspend activity.

    _____   Review potential allergens in the home environment.

Exercise 3

Virtual Hospital Activity

30 minutes

- Sign in to work at Pacific View Regional Hospital for Period of Care 3. (*Note:* If you are already in the virtual hospital from a previous exercise, click on **Leave the Floor** and then on **Restart the Program** to get to the sign-in window.)
- From the Patient List, select Patricia Newman (Room 406).
- Click on **Get Report** and read the shift report.
- Click on **Go to Nurses' Station**.
- Click on **Chart** and then on **406**.
- Click on and review the **History and Physical** and **Physician's Notes**.

1. Why has Patricia Newman been admitted to the hospital?

2. What are Patricia Newman's medical diagnoses?

3. Potential infectious causes of pneumonia include _____, _____,

   and _____.

4. Which conditions in Patricia Newman's medical history increase her risk for the development of pneumonia? Select all that apply.

   _____   Smoking

   _____   Hypertension

   _____   Osteoporosis

   _____   Social isolation

   _____   Hysterectomy

   _____   Emphysema

5. Which characteristics are associated with emphysema? Select all that apply.

   _____   Emphysema affects both men and women.

   _____   Symptoms typically begin to manifest while the patient is in the mid- to late 30s.

   _____   The disorder is characterized by changes in the alveolar walls and capillaries.

   _____   Disability often results in patients diagnosed with emphysema between the ages of 50 and 60 years.

   _____   Heredity may play a role in the development of emphysema.

• Click on and review the **Laboratory Reports**.

6. Which component of Patricia Newman's hematology test is abnormal?
   a. White blood cell (WBC) count
   b. RBC count
   c. Hgb
   d. Hct
   e. Mean corpuscular volume (MCV)
   f. Platelets

7. Review the ABG values drawn on Wednesday at 0600. Complete the chart. Indicate with an asterisk (*) any values that are abnormal.

ABG	Patricia Newman's Level	Normal Range
PaO$_2$		
O$_2$ saturation		
PaCO$_2$		
pH		

8. What inferences can be made based on the values in the previous question?

9. What is the identified cause of Patricia Newman's pneumonia?

10. Which manifestations are consistent with the type of pneumonia that Patricia Newman has? Select all that apply.

_____ Burning or searing chest pain

_____ Barking cough

_____ Stabbing chest pain

_____ Abrupt onset of symptoms

_____ Fever

• Click on and review the **Diagnostic Reports**.

11. The chest x-ray impression states that there are right middle and lower lobe infiltrates. Discuss how this manifestation takes place.

12. Identify several potential complications associated with pneumonia.

- Click on **Return to Nurses' Station** and then on **406** at the bottom of the screen.
- Review the Initial Observations.
- Click on **Take Vital Signs** and review the findings.

13. List Patricia Newman's vital signs. (*Note:* Answers will vary depending on the exact time they are taken.)

    Temperature: _____

    Heart rate: _____

    Blood pressure: _____

    Respirations: _____

- Click on **Patient Care** and then on **Physical Assessment**. Complete a systems assessment by clicking on the body system categories (yellow buttons) and body system subcategories (green buttons).

14. Identify findings from the systems assessment that are consistent with the diagnosis of pneumonia.

15. List several nursing interventions that could be implemented to improve Patricia Newman's airway clearance.

16. Cefotan has been ordered to treat Patricia Newman's pneumonia. Which is a frequent side effect associated with this medication?
    a. Oral candidiasis
    b. Nausea
    c. Vomiting
    d. Rash
    e. Pruritus
    f. Thrombophlebitis

17. Which occurrences will signal successful action by the prescribed Cefotan? Select all that apply.

    _____ Increase in RBC count

    _____ Decrease in RBC count

    _____ Reduction in temperature

    _____ Reduction in O_2 saturation

    _____ Reduction in blood pressure

    _____ Decrease in WBC count

Cardiac Disorders

Reading Assignment: Cardiac Disorders (Chapter 36)

Patient: Piya Jordan, Room 403

Objectives:

1. Review the signs and symptoms of atrial fibrillation.
2. Review the use of treatment therapies for atrial fibrillation.
3. Identify risk factors for coronary artery disease.
4. List the classifications of selected medications used in the care of cardiovascular disorders.
5. Identify dietary modifications for the patient with a cardiac disorder.

Exercise 1

Writing Activity

15 minutes

1. A patient has been diagnosed with a cardiac disorder in which the pacemaker of her heart is dysfunctional. What part of the heart is most likely implicated?
   a. The AV node
   b. The SA node
   c. The Purkinje fibers
   d. The bundle of His

2. When systole of the cardiac cycle occurs, what is happening?
   a. The right atrium is contracting.
   b. The right ventricle is contracting.
   c. The left atrium is contracting.
   d. The left ventricle is contracting.

3. There are four valves in the heart. What is their function?

4. List the four cardiac valves.

5. A patient experiencing cardiac problems has undergone testing and is found to have an elevated preload. What factor may have contributed to this phenomenon?
   a. Dehydration
   b. Hemorrhage
   c. Overhydration
   d. Venous vasodilation

6. Match each drug with its correct classification. (*Note:* Some classifications will be used more than once.)

	Drug		**Classification**
_____	Nitroglycerin	a.	Antiplatelet agent
_____	Atenolol	b.	Antianginal agent
_____	Procardia	c.	Antidysrhythmic agent
_____	Phenytoin sodium (Dilantin)		
_____	Ticlopidine (Ticlid)		
_____	Verapamil (Calan)		

7. To manage fluid retention in the patient with a cardiac condition, sodium may be restricted to

   _____ mg/day.

8. When providing dietary education to the patient with a heart condition, it is recommended that cholesterol intake be limited to what amount each day?
   a. 100 mg/day
   b. 200 mg/day
   c. 350 mg/day
   d. 400 mg/day

9. Which are risk factors for a myocardial infarction? Select all that apply.

   _____ Obesity

   _____ Diet low in fiber

   _____ History of diabetes mellitus

   _____ Smoking

   _____ Sedentary lifestyle

   _____ Hypertension

   _____ Female gender

10. Troponin levels have been drawn on a patient suspected of having suffered a myocardial infarction. Which finding is consistent with this diagnosis?
    a. Troponin levels are elevated for 1 to 2 hours after the myocardial injury.
    b. Troponin levels peak in 12 hours.
    c. Elevations in troponin levels will last for 5 to 7 days.
    d. Troponin levels begin to elevate 8 hours after the myocardial injury.

Exercise 2

Virtual Hospital Activity

45 minutes

- Sign in to work at Pacific View Regional Hospital for Period of Care 1. (*Note:* If you are already in the virtual hospital from a previous exercise, click on **Leave the Floor** and then on **Restart the Program** to get to the sign-in window.)
- From the Patient List, select Piya Jordan (Room 403).
- Click on **Get Report** and read the shift report.
- Click on **Go to Nurses' Station**.
- Click on **Chart** and then on **403**.
- Click on **History and Physical** and review Piya Jordan's history.

1. Identify any cardiac-related disorders in Piya Jordan's health history.

2. At the time of Piya Jordan's admission, had she presented with any alterations in cardiac function? Review and report the findings of her cardiac assessment at the time of her admission.

3. What were Piya Jordan's vital signs on admission?

4. Review and report any abnormality in her heart rate.

5. Briefly explain the underlying cause of Piya Jordan's cardiac condition.

6. What are signs and symptoms of this condition?

7. Which may be associated with the onset of atrial fibrillation? Select all that apply.

_____ Dehydration

_____ Myocardial infarction

_____ Mitral valve stenosis

_____ COPD

_____ Hyperthyroidism

_____ Cardiomyopathy

_____ Rheumatic heart disease

• Click on **Nursing Admission** and review.

8. What medications does Piya Jordan take at home?

- Click on **Return to Nurses' Station**.
- Click on **403** to enter Piya Jordan's room.
- Click on **Check Armband**.
- Review the **Initial Observations**.
- Click on **Take Vital Signs** and review the findings.

9. List Piya Jordan's vital signs. Are they within normal limits? If not, identify abnormalities.

- Click on **Patient Care** and then on **Physical Assessment**. Complete a chest assessment by clicking on the appropriate body system categories (yellow buttons) and body system subcategories (green buttons).

10. What equipment is being used for her cardiac monitoring?

11. What findings are consistent with atrial fibrillation?

- Click on **MAR** and then on **403**.
- Review Piya Jordan's ordered medications.

12. The physician has prescribed digoxin. To which classification does this medication belong?
    a. Cardiac glycoside
    b. Antianginal agent
    c. ACE inhibitor
    d. Anticoagulant agent

13. Which actions are attributed to digoxin therapy? Select all that apply.

    _____   Increases cardiac output

    _____   Reduces preload

    _____   Delays impulse conduction

    _____   Increases strength of myocardial contraction

    _____   Acts as a vasodilator of arteries and veins

14. Piya Jordan's prescribed dosage of digoxin is _____ IV.

15. What is the normal range for the maintenance IV dosage of digoxin daily?
    a. 0.75 to 1.5 mg
    b. 0.1 to 0.4 mg
    c. 0.5 to 2 mg
    d. 1 to 1.5 mg

16. What is the range for therapeutic digoxin levels?
    a. 0.5 to 1.0 ng/mL
    b. 0.75 to 1.25 ng/mL
    c. 0.8 to 2.0 ng/mL
    d. 1.0 to 2.35 ng/mL

- Click on **Chart** and then on **403**.
- Click and review **Laboratory Reports**.

17. Digoxin levels have been ordered for Piya Jordan. What are the ranges for the digoxin levels tested?

18. Which are considered early manifestations of digoxin toxicity? Select all that apply.

_____ Headache

_____ Anorexia

_____ Hypertension

_____ Facial pain

_____ Personality changes

_____ Weaknesses

_____ Confusion

Cardiovascular Disorders: Hypertension

Reading Assignment: Hypertension (Chapter 38)

Patient: Patricia Newman, Room 406

Objectives:

1. Define *hypertension*.
2. Discuss the risk factors for hypertension.
3. Identify the signs and symptoms of hypertension.
4. Understand nursing considerations of administering selected antihypertensive drugs.

Exercise 1

Writing Activity

15 minutes

1. Indicate whether each statement is true or false.

   a. _____ Hypertension is more common in women than in men.

   b. _____ Hypertension occurs three times as often in African Americans as in Caucasian Americans.

   c. _____ Ethnicity can affect a patient's ability to metabolize antihypertensive medications.

2. Patients having prehypertension have systolic pressures between _____ and _____ and

   diastolic pressures between _____ and _____.

3. Identify the two factors that determine blood pressure.

4. _____ _____ _____ is the force within blood vessels that the left ventricle must overcome to eject blood from the heart.

5. Which manifestation is associated with early-onset hypertension?
   a. Headaches at bedtime
   b. Headaches in the early morning
   c. Nasal congestion
   d. Blurred vision

6. A prehypertensive patient is attempting to avoid hypertension. Which interventions and/or lifestyle modifications will promote the patient's goal? Select all that apply.

   _____ Daily nonsteroidal antiinflammatory drug (NSAID) therapy

   _____ Isotonic exercise

   _____ Reduced cholesterol diet

   _____ Increased potassium intake

   _____ Relaxation therapies

7. A patient's physician is planning to use pharmacologic therapy to control a patient's blood pressure. Which statement concerning this treatment method is correct?
   a. Drug therapy should be the initial treatment for all cases of hypertension.
   b. A standardized drug regimen has been found to work well for a majority of patients.
   c. In proper drug therapy, a patient is initially treated with a number of drugs at high dosage levels, which are reduced over time as blood pressure is normalized.
   d. The goal of drug therapy is to use the smallest number of drugs at the lowest dosages in order to achieve good blood pressure control.

8. List the five most serious complications associated with hypertension.

9. What effects can antihypertensive medications have on sexual functioning?

Exercise 2

Virtual Hospital Activity

30 minutes

- Sign in to work at Pacific View Regional Hospital for Period of Care 1. (*Note:* If you are already in the virtual hospital form a previous exercise, click on **Leave the Floor** and then on **Restart the Program** to get to the sign-in window.)
- From the Patient List, select Patricia Newman (Room 406).
- Click on **Get Report** and read the shift report.
- Click on **Go to Nurses' Station**.
- Click on **Chart** and then on **406**.
- Click on and review the **History and Physical**.

1. Identify significant health concerns from Patricia Newman's medical history.

- Click on and review the **Nursing Admission**.

2. Upon admission, Patricia Newman's blood pressure was _____.

- Click on **Return to Nurses' Station**.
- Click on the **Drug** icon and review the entries for atenolol and chlorothiazide.

3. Patricia Newman takes atenolol 50 mg PO and chlorothiazide 500 mg PO daily to manage her hypertension. Identify the action or classification of each of these medications.

4. The normally recommended dosage of atenolol is _____ to _____ mg.

5. _____ Patricia Newman's prescribed dosage of atenolol is within recommended limits. (True/False)

6. Which manifestations are side effects associated with atenolol? Select all that apply.

_____ Cold extremities

_____ Constipation

_____ Diarrhea

_____ Nausea

_____ Headache

_____ Impotence

7. Chlorothiazide is associated with excretion of which electrolytes? Select all that apply.

_____ Sodium

_____ Phosphorus

_____ Potassium

_____ Zinc

_____ Calcium

_____ Magnesium

_____ Chloride

8. The physician has ordered atenolol and chlorothiazide. Describe the relationship between the two medications.

9. Identify several nursing considerations for Patricia Newman in relation to the medications prescribed to manage her hypertension.

• Click on **Return to Nurses' Station**.
• Click on **Chart** and then on **406**.
• Click on and review the **Laboratory Reports**.

10. Patricia Newman's potassium level is 3.2 mEq/L. Which foods should be added to her diet to manage these levels? Select all that apply.

    _____ Broccoli

    _____ Lettuce

    _____ Apricots

    _____ Apples

    _____ Blueberries

    _____ Prunes

11. A normal potassium level is between _____ and _____ mEq/L.

12. To which hypertension risk group does Patricia Newman belong?
    a. Group A
    b. Group B
    c. Group C

13. Which best describes Patricia Newman's hypertension?
    a. Primary
    b. Secondary
    c. Tertiary

14. Several risk factors for developing hypertension are listed below. Which of these risk factors apply to Patricia Newman? Select all that apply.

    _____ Dyslipidemia

    _____ Atherosclerosis

    _____ Diabetes mellitus

    _____ Cigarette smoking

    _____ Aging

    _____ Gender

    _____ Obesity

    _____ Sedentary lifestyle

Digestive Tract Disorders

Reading Assignment: Upper Digestive Tract Disorders (Chapter 39)
Lower Digestive Tract Disorders (Chapter 40)

Patient: Piya Jordan, Room 403

Objectives:

1. Identify nursing responsibilities in caring for patients undergoing diagnostic tests and procedures for digestive tract disorders.

2. List data to be included in the nursing assessment of a patient with a digestive tract disorder.

3. Describe nursing care of patients with gastrointestinal (GI) intubation and decompression, tube feedings, total parenteral nutrition, digestive tract surgery, and drug therapy for digestive tract disorders.

4. Describe the pathophysiology, signs and symptoms, complications, and medical treatment of selected digestive tract disorders.

Exercise 1

Writing Activity

45 minutes

1. The functions of the digestive tract are _____, _____,

   _____ of nutrients, and _____ of wastes.

2. Match each GI structure with the corresponding digestive function.

GI Structure	Digestive Function
_____ Mouth	a. No known function
_____ Colon	b. Closes when food is swallowed to prevent aspiration
_____ Epiglottis	c. Secretes bile for the emulsification of fat
_____ Esophagus	d. Mixes food with saliva
_____ Pancreatic duct	e. Finishes digestion and absorption of chyme across a smaller number of villi, especially at the distal end
_____ Ilium	
_____ Appendix	f. Reabsorbs water and electrolytes and prepares waste for excretion
_____ Liver	g. Transports food bolus from mouth to stomach
_____ Pyloric sphincter	h. Collects pancreatic enzymes and transports them to the duodenum
	i. Prevents backflow of alkaline intestinal contents into the stomach

3. Which techniques should the nurse include when examining the abdomen? Select all that apply.

   _____ The patient should be in semi-Fowler position.

   _____ The patient should be supine.

   _____ The patient's knees should be flat.

   _____ The patient's knees should be slightly flexed.

   _____ The patient's abdomen should be thought of as divided into four quadrants.

4. _____ When assessing for bowel sounds, the nurse should listen for at least 1 minute before recording bowel sounds as absent. (True/False)

5. When caring for the patient who has had a gastroscopy performed, the nurse should include which elements in the plan of care?
   a. Monitor stools for at least 2 days for the passage of white stools.
   b. Administer laxatives.
   c. Encourage fluid intake to flush the patient's system.
   d. Continue to administer nothing by mouth (NPO) until gag reflex returns.

6. A nurse is providing information for a patient scheduled to have stool specimens collected to test for the presence of occult blood. Which food items may interfere with the test results? Select all that apply.

   _____ Red meat

   _____ Poultry

   _____ Milk

   _____ Orange juice

   _____ Steroids

7. When a nurse is planning food options for a patient who has difficulty swallowing, which foods should be included? Select all that apply.

   _____ Lukewarm foods

   _____ Cold foods

   _____ Mildly sweetened foods

   _____ Pureed foods

   _____ Moist pasta

8. Which events can increase the body's nutritional needs? Select all that apply.

   _____ Infection

   _____ Fever

   _____ Rest

   _____ Stress

   _____ Trauma

9. A patient suspected of having Crohn's disease is being educated about an upcoming fecal fat test. What information should be provided to the patient?
   a. Adhere to a restricted fat diet for 1 week before the test
   b. Administer a Fleet enema the day before the test
   c. NPO status after midnight of the night before the test
   d. Refrigerate the stool specimen after collection
   e. Adhere to a 60-gram fat diet for 3 to 6 days before the test

10. To reduce the risk for aspiration after a tube feeding, a nurse should keep the head of a patient's bed elevated for how long?
    a. 15 minutes
    b. 30 minutes
    c. 1 hour
    d. 90 minutes

11. In which populations is inherited lactase deficiency prevalent? Select all that apply.

    _____ European

    _____ African American

    _____ South American

    _____ Mediterranean

    _____ Asian

12. A patient underwent a gastric surgical procedure in which the end of the stomach was connected to the duodenum. What terms are used to refer to this procedure?
    a. Total gastrectomy
    b. Modified gastrectomy
    c. Billroth I procedure
    d. Billroth II procedure

13. Compare and contrast gastric and duodenal ulcers.

Characteristics	Gastric Ulcer	Duodenal Ulcer
Location		
Population		
Manifestations		

14. Most ulcers are caused by _____ _____.

15. Match each GI disorder with its correct description.

GI Disorder

_____ Gastroesophageal reflux disease (GERD)

_____ Candidiasis

_____ Gastritis

_____ Irritable bowel syndrome

_____ Ulcerative colitis

_____ Crohn's disease

_____ Diverticulosis

Description

a. Presence of herniations in the muscular layers of the colon

b. An inflammatory condition of the GI tract causing a cobblestone-like appearance in the mucosa

c. Episodic bowel dysfunction characterized by intestinal pain, disturbed defecation, or abdominal distention

d. Presence of abscesses on the colon mucosa and submucosa causing drainage, sloughing, and subsequent ulcerations

e. Backflow of stomach acid into the esophagus

f. Fungal infection presenting as white patches on the mucous membranes

g. Inflammation of the lining of the stomach

16. Match each drug with the corresponding use and/or action.

Drug

_____ Diphenoxylate hydrochloride (HCl) (Lomotil)

_____ Metoclopramide (Reglan)

_____ Sulfasalazine (Azulfidine)

_____ Nystatin (Mycostatin)

_____ Sucralfate (Carafate)

_____ Cimetidine (Tagamet)

_____ Promethazine HCl (Phenergan)

Use/Action

a. Interacts with acid to form a protective gel that coats ulcer surface and promotes healing

b. Antiinfective used to manage ulcerative colitis

c. Decreases intestinal motility

d. Reduces secretion of gastric acid and promotes healing of ulcers

e. Antifungal

f. Increases the speed of gastric emptying into the small intestine

g. Prevents and treats nausea

Exercise 2

Virtual Hospital Activity

45 minutes

- Sign in to work at Pacific View Regional Hospital for Period of Care 2. (*Note:* If you are already in the virtual hospital from a previous exercise, click on **Leave the Floor** and then on **Restart the Program** to get to the sign-in window.)
- From the Patient List, select Piya Jordan (Room 403).
- Click on **Get Report** and read the shift report.
- Click on **Go to Nurses' Station** and then on **403** at the bottom of the screen.
- Click on **Patient Care** and then on **Nurse-Client Interactions**.
- Select and view the video titled **1115: Interventions—Nausea, Blood**. (*Note:* Check the virtual clock to see whether enough time has elapsed. You can use the fast-forward feature to advance the time by 2-minute intervals if the video is not yet available. Then click again on **Patient Care** and **Nurse-Client Interactions** to refresh the screen.)

1. Based on your review of the shift report and the video, which care factors appear to be of the highest priority?

- Click on **Chart** and then on **403**.
- Click on and review the **History and Physical** and **Nursing Admission**.

2. Why did Piya Jordan initially seek care?

- Click on **Emergency Department** and review the Emergency Department physician's notes.

3. What was Piya Jordan's diagnosis after the medical examination in the Emergency Department?

4. An intestinal obstruction can be caused by a mass or by a number of other factors. List several of these factors.

5. Vomiting associated with an intestinal obstruction can lead to fluid and electrolyte imbalances and

   _____ _____.

6. Is Piya Jordan's intestinal obstruction considered mechanical or nonmechanical?

• Click on and review the **Diagnostic Reports**.

7. Which diagnostic tests were used to determine the underlying cause of Piya Jordan's condition? Select all that apply.

   _____ Computed tomography (CT) scan of the abdomen

   _____ Kidney-ureter-bladder x-ray (KUB)

   _____ Chest x-ray

   _____ Electrocardiogram (ECG)

   _____ Endoscopy

   _____ Colonoscopy

• Click on and review the **Surgical Reports**.

8. What were Piya Jordan's postoperative diagnoses?

9. Which best describes the surgical procedure performed on Piya Jordan?
   a. Removal of the entire small intestine
   b. Removal of the entire large intestine
   c. Removal of the distal portion of the stomach and small intestine
   d. Removal of a portion of the large intestine

10. Which portion of Piya Jordan's intestine was involved in the obstruction?

11. Which factors put an individual at increased risk for the development of colorectal cancer? Select all that apply.

   _____   History of ulcerative colitis

   _____   History of Crohn's disease

   _____   History of hiatal hernia

   _____   High-fat diet

   _____   High-fiber diet

   _____   Family history of colorectal cancer

12. Where are the majority of colorectal cancers located?

- Click on **Return to Room 403**.
- Click on **Take Vital Signs**.
- Review the Initial Observations.
- Click on and review the **Clinical Alerts**.
- Click on **Patient Care** and then on **Physical Assessment**. Complete a systems assessment by clicking on the body system categories (yellow buttons) and body system subcategories (green buttons).

13. Piya Jordan's assessment findings reflect the greatest potential for development of postoperative complications in which body systems?
   a. Respiratory
   b. Renal
   c. Integumentary
   d. Reproductive
   e. Neurologic

14. Management and care of a patient who has had GI surgery frequently includes the placement of a nasogastric (NG) tube. An NG tube has a variety of functions. Match each NG function with the corresponding description.

Function	Description
_____ Decompression	a. Irrigation of the stomach; used in cases of active bleeding, poisoning, or gastric dilation
_____ Feeding	b. Removal of secretions and gases from the GI tract
_____ Compression	c. Internal application of pressure by means of an inflated balloon to prevent internal GI hemorrhage
_____ Lavage	d. Instillation of liquid supplements into the stomach

15. Why was Piya Jordan's NG tube inserted?

16. Discuss responsibilities of the nurse regarding the care and management of Piya Jordan's NG tube.

• Click on **EPR** and then on **Login**.
• Select **403** from the Patient drop-down menu and **Intake and Output** from the Category drop-down menu. Use the arrows at the bottom of the screen to view all entries.

17. What is the total amount of drainage from Piya Jordan's NG tube?

18. _____ The absence of bowel sounds at this stage of Piya Jordan's recovery is normal. (True/False)

19. When the nurse performs an assessment on Piya Jordan's abdomen, in what order should the tools of observation occur?

Tool of Assessment	**Order of Occurrence**
_____ Palpation	a. First
_____ Inspection	b. Second
_____ Percussion	c. Third
_____ Auscultation	d. Fourth

Connective Tissue Disorders

Reading Assignment: Connective Tissue Disorders (Chapter 43)
Fractures (Chapter 44)

Patients: Harry George, Room 401
Clarence Hughes, Room 404

Objectives:

1. Describe the functions of connective tissue.

2. Describe the characteristics and prevalence of connective tissue disorders.

3. Describe the diagnostic tests and procedures used for assessing connective tissue disorders.

4. Discuss drugs used to treat connective tissue disorders.

5. Discuss the care of the patient with osteomyelitis.

6. Identify risk factors for osteoporosis.

7. Recognize complications associated with osteoporosis.

8. Discuss treatment plans for the management of osteoporosis.

Exercise 1

Writing Activity

30 minutes

1. Indicate whether each statement is true or false.

   a. _____ Rheumatoid disorders affect women more frequently than men.

   b. _____ Drug therapy can provide a cure for osteoarthritis.

   c. _____ To avoid addiction, it is best for patients affected by osteoarthritis to take medications only when pain is present.

2. _____ _____ bind structures together, providing support for individual organs and a framework for the body as a whole.

3. When performing an assessment of the musculoskeletal system, the nurse must listen for a crackling

   sound known as _____.

4. List the age-related changes of connective tissues.

5. When a patient is being prepared for a C-reactive protein test, which instructions should be included?
   a. Fast for 8 hours before the test.
   b. Obtain a clean-catch, midstream urine specimen.
   c. Restrict red meat intake on the day before the test.
   d. Restrict fluids and food for 4 hours before the test.

6. When a nurse is preparing a patient for an arthrography, which steps must be completed? Select all that apply.

   _____ Assess the patient for allergy to the contrast agent.

   _____ Assess the patient for allergy to seafood.

   _____ Advise the patient that needle insertion may cause discomfort.

   _____ Administer a Fleet enema for patient.

   _____ Instruct the patient that swelling at the insertion site may be experienced.

7. Which diagnostic test would most likely be used to identify masses or fluid in soft tissue?
   a. Ultrasonography
   b. Tomography
   c. Nuclear scintigraphy
   d. Diskography

8. Match each drug with its corresponding classification and/or use.

Drug	**Classification/Use**
_____ Naproxen (Naprosyn)	a. Indole analogue
_____ Celecoxib (Celebrex)	b. First-generation nonsteroidal antiinflammatory drug (NSAID)
_____ Indomethacin (Indocin)	c. Second-generation NSAID; COX-2 inhibitor
_____ Methotrexate (Folex)	d. Used in the treatment of gout
_____ Etanercept (Enbrel)	e. Disease-modifying antirheumatic drug (DMARD)
_____ Allopurinol (Zyloprim)	f. Antiarthritic, biologic response modifiers

9. Rheumatoid arthritis is most common in people between _____ and _____ years of age.

10. Which factors are possible causes of rheumatoid arthritis? Select all that apply.

    _____ Autoimmune response

    _____ Viral links

    _____ Genetic predisposition

    _____ Reproductive history

    _____ Hormonal factors

    _____ Breastfeeding

    _____ History of osteoarthritis

11. Which clinical manifestations are associated with rheumatoid arthritis? Select all that apply.

    _____ Pain aggravated by movement

    _____ Pain that eases within 20 to 30 minutes of rising in the morning

    _____ Weakness

    _____ Weight gain

    _____ Bilateral joint changes

    _____ Muscle aches and tenderness

12. Gout is a systemic disease characterized by deposits of _____

_____ in the joints and other body tissues.

13. Which factors are associated with gout? Select all that apply.

_____ Genetic links

_____ Malnutrition

_____ Alcohol consumption

_____ Hypouricemia

_____ Thiazide diuretics

14. Which medication may be prescribed by the physician to treat an episode of gout?
    a. Colchicine
    b. Indomethacin
    c. Corticotropin
    d. Sulfa compounds
    e. Allopurinol

15. When planning the diet of a patient with gout, the nurse should exclude which foods? Select all that apply.

_____ Leafy green vegetables

_____ Gravy

_____ Sardines

_____ Organ meats

_____ Citrus fruits

16. _____ _____ _____ is a systemic disorder characterized by hardening of the skin.

Exercise 2

Virtual Hospital Activity

45 minutes

- Sign in to work at Pacific View Regional Hospital for Period of Care 1. (*Note:* If you are already in the virtual hospital from a previous exercise, click on **Leave the Floor** and then on **Restart the Program** to get to the sign-in window.)
- From the Patient List, select Harry George (Room 401).
- Click on **Get Report** and read the shift report.
- Click on **Go to Nurses' Station**.
- Click on **Chart** and then on **401**.
- Click on and review the **Nursing Admission**, **History and Physical**, and **Physician's Notes**.

1. Why has Harry George sought medical care?

2. After a medical examination, what diagnoses have been identified?

3. What factors in Harry George's medical and social history put him at risk for the development of osteomyelitis?

4. Which clinical manifestations are associated with osteomyelitis? Select all that apply.

_____ Generalized pain

_____ Erythremia in surrounding tissues

_____ Wound drainage

_____ Elevated temperature

_____ Chills

- Click on and review the **Physician's Orders**.
- Click on and review the **Laboratory Reports** and **Diagnostic Reports**.

5. Which tests were ordered specifically to confirm the diagnosis of osteomyelitis? Select all that apply.

_____ Complete blood count (CBC)

_____ Urinalysis

_____ Albumin levels

_____ Hemoglobin A_{1C}

_____ Blood alcohol levels

_____ Folic acid levels

_____ Bone scan

_____ X-ray of left foot

_____ Chest x-ray

6. Which laboratory values for Harry George were abnormal? Select all that apply.

_____ Red blood cell (RBC) count

_____ White blood cell (WBC) count

_____ Hemoglobin (Hgb)

_____ Hematocrit (Hct)

_____ Platelets

_____ Neutrophils segmented (segs)

_____ Neutrophils bands

_____ Lymphocytes

_____ Monocytes

_____ Eosinophils

_____ Basophils

7. Which statement regarding Harry George's erythrocyte sedimentation rate (ESR) is correct?
   a. The ESR is decreased as a result of the infection.
   b. The ESR is increased as a result of the infection.
   c. Harry George's diabetes suppresses the ESR value.
   d. Patients with diabetes have a natural elevation in ESR.

8. Discuss the results of Harry George's x-ray and bone scan.

9. _____ _____ was identified as the pathogen responsible for Harry George's infection.

10. _____ Harry George also has tested positive for septicemia. (True/False)

11. In addition to medications, what other interventions have been ordered to manage Harry George's osteomyelitis?

12. What consultations have been ordered to assist in the care of Harry George's osteomyelitis?

- Click on **Return to Nurses' Station** and then on **401** at the bottom of the screen.
- Click on **Take Vital Signs**.
- Review the Initial Observations.
- Click on and review the **Clinical Alerts**.

13. Record Harry George's vital signs below. (*Note:* Findings will vary depending on exact time vital signs are taken.)

Temperature: _____

Heart rate: _____

Respiratory rate: _____

Blood pressure: _____

Pain level: _____

Oxygen saturation (SpO$_2$): _____

14. Are any of Harry George's vital signs consistent with the presence of an infection? If so, which ones?

- Click on **Patient Care** and then on **Physical Assessment**. Complete a head-to-toe assessment by clicking on the body system categories (yellow buttons) and body system subcategories (green buttons).

15. What findings from the assessment of Harry George's lower extremities are consistent with the diagnosis of osteomyelitis?

- Click on **MAR** and then on tab **401**.
- Review the medications ordered for Harry George.

16. Which medications have been ordered to manage Harry George's infection? Select all that apply. (*Hint:* Refer to the Drug Guide if needed).

_____ Gentamicin 20 mg IV

_____ Thiamine 100 mg PO/IM

_____ Cefotaxime 2 g IV

_____ Phenytoin sodium 100 mg IV

_____ Aluminum hydroxide with magnesium 30 mL

17. Harry George was last medicated for pain at _____. The next time that he will be able to receive

analgesics is _____.

18. Once administered, how long will it take for the analgesic to take effect?
    a. 10 to 15 minutes
    b. 15 to 30 minutes
    c. 30 minutes
    d. 1 hour

19. What is the anticipated duration of Harry George's analgesic?
    a. 1 to 2 hours
    b. 2 to 3 hours
    c. 3 to 4 hours
    d. 4 to 5 hours

Exercise 3

Virtual Hospital Activity

45 minutes

- Sign in to work at Pacific View Regional Hospital for Period of Care 1. (*Note:* If you are already in the virtual hospital from a previous exercise, click on **Leave the Floor** and then on **Restart the Program** to get to the sign-in window.)
- From the Patient List, select Clarence Hughes (Room 404).
- Click on **Get Report** and read the shift report.
- Click on **Go to Nurses' Station** and then on **404** at the bottom of the screen.
- Review the Initial Observations.
- Click on **Chart** and then on **404**.
- Click on and review the **History and Physical**, **Nursing Admission**, and **Physician's Notes**.

1. Why has Clarence Hughes been admitted to the hospital?

2. Clarence Hughes has degenerative joint disease. This condition is also known as

   _____.

3. Which populations are at an increased risk for the development of osteoarthritis? Select all that apply.

   _____ Small-framed patients

   _____ Obese patients

   _____ Older patients

   _____ Individuals whose occupations require repetitive joint movements

   _____ Women of childbearing age

   _____ Individuals with diabetes

4. Which joints are most likely to be affected by osteoarthritis?

5. According to Clarence Hughes' admission data, he has a history of an arthroscopy. Which statement concerning this procedure is most correct?
   a. The arthroscopy involves obtaining a specimen of muscle tissue for study.
   b. The arthroscopy allows the visualization of the joint cavity.
   c. After the arthroscopy there is no need to limit activity.
   d. The arthroscopy provides a definitive diagnosis for inflammatory connective tissue diseases.

6. Which clinical manifestation is associated with osteoarthritis?
   a. Joint pain in the morning upon arising
   b. Bilateral joint involvement
   c. Joint enlargement
   d. Systemic involvement

7. Clarence Hughes has been taking celecoxib 100 mg PO BID to manage his osteoarthritis. Which terms accurately describe this medication? Select all that apply.

   _____ Antiinflammatory

   _____ Used to manage allergic conditions

   _____ Inhibits platelet aggregation (clumping)

   _____ Antipyretic

   _____ Analgesic

• Click on and review the **Surgical Reports**.

8. What surgical procedure was completed to manage Clarence Hughes' condition?

9. _____ Joint replacement is avoided in patients younger than 50 years. (True/False)

10. The life expectancy of a modern prosthesis is _____ years.

- Click on **Return to Room 404**.
- Click on **Take Vital Signs**.

11. _____ Clarence Hughes' vital signs are within normal limits. (True/False)

- Review the Initial Observations.
- Click on and review the **Clinical Alerts**.
- Click on **Patient Care** and then on **Physical Assessment**. Complete a systems assessment by clicking on the body system categories (yellow buttons) and body system subcategories (green buttons).

12. Which of Clarence Hughes' care needs are of the highest priority?

13. Which interventions may be used to assist Clarence Hughes in the management of his postoperative pain? Select all that apply.

_____ Heating pad

_____ Massage

_____ Relaxation techniques

_____ Analgesics

_____ Imagery

14. The physician has ordered the use of a continuous passive motion (CPM) machine. What is the rationale for the use of this equipment? Select all that apply.

_____ To reduce the formation of scar tissue

_____ To promote mobility

_____ To manage postoperative pain

_____ To reduce the risk for infection

_____ To lengthen the life expectancy of the prosthetic device

15. _____ The physician has ordered Clarence Hughes to remain in bed for the first postoperative day. (True/False)

16. List several potential postoperative complications for the patient who has had joint replacement surgery.

- Click on MAR and then on tab **404**.

17. Which medication was ordered to manage Clarence Hughes' pain?
    a. Acetaminophen 650 mg PO every 6 hours
    b. Temazepam 15 mg PO
    c. Oxycodone with acetaminophen 1 to 2 tablets PO every 4 hours
    d. Enoxaparin 30 mg subQ every 12 hours

Exercise 4

Virtual Hospital Activity

45 minutes

- Sign in to work at Pacific View Regional Hospital for Period of Care 2. (*Note:* If you are already in the virtual hospital from a previous exercise, click on **Leave the Floor** and then on **Restart the Program** to get to the sign-in window.)
- From the Patient List, select Patricia Newman (Room 406).
- Click on **Get Report** and read the shift report.
- Click on **Go to Nurses' Station**.
- Click on **Chart** and then on **404**.
- Click on and review the **History and Physical**.

1. What are Patricia Newman's medical diagnoses?

2. What was her chief medical complaint at the time of admission?

3. Patricia Newman has a history of osteoporosis. Describe this condition.

4. A bone density test may be used to assess bone mass. On what sites may this test be performed? Select all that apply.

_____ Finger

_____ Ulna

_____ Radius

_____ Femur

_____ Heel

5. What are potential signs and symptoms of osteoporosis?

6. Which parts of Patricia Newman's body are at the highest risk for fracture related to osteoporosis?

7. Between _____% and _____% of bone mass is lost before it can be visualized by radiologic studies.

8. What factors are noted in Patricia Newman's health history that are risk factors for the development of osteoporosis?

• Click and review **Physician's Orders** in the chart.

9. Review the medications prescribed for Patricia Newman. Which medications prescribed may have an impact on osteoporosis?

10. What impact will each of the medications you identified in the preceding question have on Patricia Newman's osteoporosis?

Endocrine Disorders: Diabetes Mellitus and Hypoglycemia

Reading Assignment: Diabetes Mellitus and Hypoglycemia (Chapter 48)

Patient: Harry George, Room 401

Objectives:

1. Describe the role of insulin in the body.

2. Explain the pathophysiology of diabetes mellitus and hypoglycemia.

3. Describe the signs and symptoms of diabetes mellitus and hypoglycemia.

4. Explain tests and procedures used to diagnose diabetes mellitus and hypoglycemia.

5. Discuss the treatment of diabetes mellitus and hypoglycemia.

6. Explain the differences between type 1 and type 2 diabetes mellitus.

7. Describe the complications of diabetes mellitus.

Exercise 1

Writing Activity

45 minutes

1. _____% of the total U.S. population has diabetes mellitus.

2. Insulin is a hormone produced by the _____ _____ in the

   _____ of _____.

3. A nurse is reviewing fasting glucose levels in a patient. Which values are considered normal ranges?
   a. 60 to 95 mg/L
   b. 70 to 100 mg/L
   c. 75 to 110 mg/L
   d. 80 to 110 mg/L

4. Indicate whether each statement is true or false.

   a. _____   Most people with diabetes have no genetic predisposition.

   b. _____   Type 2 diabetes mellitus may be controlled by diet and exercise alone.

   c. _____   The risk for diabetic nephropathy is greater for Caucasians than for Mexican
                   Americans.

5. Which statements correctly describe the presence of insulin in the body? Select all that apply.

   _____   Insulin increases the transport of glucose into the resting muscle cell.

   _____   Insulin stimulates the conversion of glycogen to glucose.

   _____   Insulin promotes fatty acid synthesis.

   _____   Insulin inhibits the conversion of protein into glucose.

   _____   Insulin halts the storage of proteins.

6. _____ _____ _____ is diagnosed when a
   pregnant woman is found to have glucose intolerance for the first time.

7. Which are risk factors for the development of type 2 diabetes mellitus? Select all that apply.

_____   Underweight

_____   Sedentary lifestyle

_____   Age 30 and younger

_____   History of delivering infant weighing more than 10 lb

_____   African American

_____   Latin American/Hispanic

8. Identify at least three long-term complications associated with diabetes mellitus.

9. Which instructions should be incorporated into a foot care teaching plan for a patient with diabetes? Select all that apply.

_____   Check feet daily.

_____   Use heating pads instead of electric blankets for discomforts of the feet and legs.

_____   Remove corns and calluses weekly.

_____   Wear shoes without stockings to promote ventilation.

_____   Wash feet daily.

_____   Use lotion daily.

10. Diabetic ketoacidosis (DKA) is an emergency medical condition caused by an absolute absence of

_____ .

11. When providing care to a patient with diabetes, it is necessary to assess for the use of herbal supplements that may affect blood glucose levels. Which supplement may reduce the blood glucose level?
    a. Onion
    b. Dill weed
    c. Parsley
    d. Cinnamon

12. During ketoacidosis, the body breaks down _____ for energy.

13. Which electrolyte is the primary concern in the management of diabetic ketoacidosis?
    a. Sodium
    b. Potassium
    c. Chloride
    d. Phosphorus
    e. Magnesium

14. Which should be included in preparation for and performance of an oral glucose tolerance test (OGTT)? Select all that apply.

    _____ The patient should consume 300 to 500 grams of carbohydrates for 3 days before the test.

    _____ The patient must remain status nothing by mouth (NPO) after midnight before the test.

    _____ The patient is given any sweet drink before a blood specimen is drawn.

    _____ The OGTT drink should be served cold to increase its appeal.

    _____ The test can be ordered for 3- or 5-hour intervals.

15. _____ Exercise is a successful means of reducing serum glucose levels greater than 300 mg/L. (True/False)

16. _____ intake may be necessary during prolonged exercise.

17. Match each type of insulin with the corresponding onset of action after administration.

	Type of Insulin	Onset of Action After Administration
_____	Lantus	a. Less than 15 minutes
_____	Humalog	b. 30 minutes to 1 hour
_____	NPH	c. 1 to 2 hours
_____	Regular	d. 2 to 4 hours
_____	Ultralente	e. 4 to 8 hours

18. Most available insulin is U/_____.

19. Which insulin can be administered intravenously?
    a. Regulat
    b. Lantus
    c. NPH
    d. Humalog

20. _____ Lantus cannot be mixed with other types of insulin. (True/False)

21. A nurse is caring for a patient experiencing minor hypoglycemia. Which intervention is the best initial action for the nurse to take?
    a. Notifying the physician
    b. Administering an IV bolus of glucose solution
    c. Providing the patient with cheese, crackers, and a glass of milk
    d. Providing the patient with a nutritional source containing 20 g of carbohydrate
    e. Offering the patient a glass of fruit juice

Exercise 2

Virtual Hospital Activity

45 minutes

- Sign into work at Pacific View Regional Hospital for Period of Care 1. (*Note:* If you are already in the virtual hospital from a previous exercise, click on **Leave the Floor** and then on **Restart the Program** to get to the sign-in window.)
- From the Patient List, select Harry George (Room 401).
- Click on **Get Report** and read the shift report.
- Click on **Go to Nurses' Station**.
- Click on **Chart** and then on **401**.
- Click on and review the **Emergency Department** record.

1. What is Harry George's chief complaint upon arrival to the Emergency Department?

2. When he arrived at the Emergency Department, Harry George's blood glucose level was _____.

3. Which type of diabetes does Harry George have?
    a. Gestational diabetes
    b. Type 1 diabetes mellitus
    c. Type 2 diabetes mellitus
    d. Pre-diabetes

4. At 1700 the Emergency Department nurse administered 10 units of regular insulin subcutaneously. What is the anticipated time of onset for the insulin?
    a. 1715
    b. 1730
    c. 1900
    d. 1930

5. Peak action of the insulin administered to Harry George will take place between _____ and

    _____.

6. The insulin administered to Harry George will demonstrate effectiveness until _____ to

    _____.

7. What type of insulin was administered to Harry George?
   a. Rapid-acting
   b. Short-acting
   c. Intermediate-acting
   d. Long-acting

• Click on and review the **Physician's Orders**.

8. The physician has ordered a(n) _____ ADA diet.

9. In this diet, what percentage of calories should come from protein?
   a. 5% to 10%
   b. 10% to 20%
   c. 25% to 30%
   d. 30% to 35%

10. What is the recommended limit for sodium intake in the daily diet for Harry George?
    a. 1,500 mg/day
    b. 2,000 mg/day
    c. 2,500 mg/day
    d. 3,000 mg/day

11. What is the schedule of blood glucose checks that the physician has ordered for Harry George?

12. The physician has ordered the use of a sliding scale for Harry George's insulin coverage. Discuss the use of a sliding scale.

13. In the event Harry George's blood glucose level is less than 150 mg/dL, would his oral hypoglycemic medication be withheld? Provide a rationale for your response.

14. What impact can illness have on Harry George's diabetes?

15. Insulin dosages are based on the total grams of _____ to be ingested.

- Click on **Return to Nurses' Station** and then on **401** at the bottom of the screen.
- Click on **Take Vital Signs** and review the findings.
- Review the Initial Observations.
- Click on and review the **Clinical Alerts**.

16. Harry George's fasting blood glucose at 0730 was _____.

- Click on **MAR** and then on tab **401**.
- Review the medications ordered for Harry George.

17. According to the sliding scale outlined in the Physician's Orders, Harry George should receive

    _____ units of insulin.

18. What oral medication has been ordered to manage Harry George's diabetes?

19. The medication identified in the preceding question belongs to which classification?
    a. Sulfonylureas
    b. Meglitinides
    c. D-phenylalanines
    d. Biguanides
    e. Alpha-glucosidase inhibitors
    f. Thiazolidinediones

20. How does the medication you identified in the preceding question work?
    a. Promotes insulin secretion by the pancreas
    b. Decreases glucose production in the liver and increasing glucose uptake by muscle
    c. Inhibits carbohydrate digestion and absorption
    d. Decreases insulin resistance

21. When administering insulin, the nurse will rotate sites. Site rotation will prevent

    _____ and _____.

22. Harry George is an alcoholic. During which time period after alcohol ingestion is hypoglycemia at the greatest risk?
    a. 4 to 6 hours
    b. 24 hours
    c. 6 to 36 hours
    d. 48 hours

Mental Health and Illness

Reading Assignment: Psychologic Responses to Illness (Chapter 55)
Psychiatric Disorders (Chapter 56)

Patient: Jacquline Catanazaro, Room 402

Objectives:

1. Define *mental health*.

2. Discuss how age, cultural beliefs, and spiritual beliefs affect an individual's ability to cope with illness.

3. Identify some basic coping strategies (defense mechanisms).

4. Identify selected medications used to manage mental illness.

Exercise 1

Writing Activity

30 minutes

1. The _____ _____ includes the biologic and physiologic aspects of a person.

2. The cognitive dimension involves the individual's ability to _____

   _____, _____ _____, and

   _____ _____.

3. List several factors that can affect an individual's ability to cope with illness.

4. After a stressful day at work, a man comes home and harshly disciplines his children. Which defense mechanism is being demonstrated?
   a. Identification
   b. Isolation
   c. Displacement
   d. Projection

5. After being sexually assaulted, the victim does not recall the events of the assault. This is reflective of which defense mechanism?
   a. Repression
   b. Regression
   c. Projection
   d. Denial

6. Which purposes are associated with a therapeutic relationship (as opposed to a social relationship)? Select all that apply.

   _____   It is mutually beneficial for all parties involved.

   _____   It develops purposefully.

   _____   Participants are not formally responsible for evaluating the interaction.

   _____   The relationship has clear boundaries.

   _____   The focus is on the personal and emotional needs of those involved.

7. _____ is a sustained feeling state or emotion that a person experiences in several aspects of life.

8. The external presentation of a person's feeling state and emotional responsiveness is referred to as the

   _____.

9. If a patient reports seeing rats crawling on his bed, what is the appropriate term for this phenomena?
   a. Illusion
   b. Dream
   c. Delusion
   d. Internal stimuli

10. _____ A patient is seen repeatedly washing her hands. This action is referred to as an obsession. (True/False)

11. The patient who is fearful to leave home has which condition?
    a. Agoraphobia
    b. Panic disorder
    c. Obsessive-compulsive disorder
    d. Posttraumatic stress disorder (PTSD)

12. A patient demonstrates a change in self-awareness. Which characteristic associated with acute stress disorder is being manifested?
    a. Derealization
    b. Depersonalization
    c. Dissociative amnesia
    d. Depression

13. Indicate whether each statement is true or false.

    a. _____ A somatoform disorder involves the appearance of physical symptoms with only minor physiologic dysfunction.

    b. _____ After experiencing a traumatic assault, a woman becomes unable to walk. This is an example of a panic disorder.

    c. _____ St. John's wort is commonly used to relieve depression.

14. In a _____ disorder, the symptoms are usually neurologic and occur in response to some threatening or traumatic event.

Exercise 2

Virtual Hospital Activity

45 minutes

- Sign in to work at Pacific View Regional Hospital for Period of Care 2. (*Note:* If you are already in the virtual hospital form a previous exercise, click on **Leave the Floor** and then on **Restart the Program** to get to the sign-in window.)
- From the Patient List, select Jacquline Catanazaro (Room 402).
- Click on **Get Report** and read the shift report.

1. Describe the psychologic behaviors documented in the shift report.

2. Jacquline Catanazaro is experiencing anxiety. What impact can this have on her respiratory distress?

- Click on **Go to Nurses' Station**.
- Click on **Chart** and then on **402**.
- Click on and review the **Emergency Department** record.

3. According to the Emergency Department record, Jacquline Catanazaro has not been taking her

   prescribed schizophrenia medications for _____ days, and she has not been taking her asthma

   medications for _____ days.

- Click on and review the **Physician's Orders**.

4. What consultations have been ordered by the physician to assist Jacquline Catanazaro?

- Click on and review the **Consultations**.

5. When was Jacquline Catanazaro diagnosed with schizophrenia?

6. Schizophrenia refers to a chronic disorder in which the patient's ability to interpret the environment is

   impaired by _____.

7. Indicate whether each statement is true or false.

   a. _____ The time of life in which Jacquline Catanazaro was diagnosed with schizophrenia is
   typical of the disorder.

   b. _____ After recovery from an acute exacerbation of schizophrenia, a patient may not return to
   the level of functioning experienced before the event.

8. What manifestations are associated with psychotic symptoms of schizophrenia?

9. Discuss the plan outlined by the psychiatrist.

• Click on and review the **Nursing Admission**.

10. _____ Jacquline Catanazaro has a positive family history of mental illness. (True/False)

11. To what does Jacquline Catanazaro attribute her lack of compliance with her prescribed medications?
    a. Financial concerns
    b. Belief that the medications are dangerous for her
    c. Concerns about the side effects of the medications on her weight
    d. Inability to remember to take medications

12. Where does the majority of Jacquline Catanazaro's social support come from?
    a. Her ex-husbands
    b. Her sister
    c. Her adult children
    d. Her parents

13. Discuss Jacquline Catanazaro's use of alcohol and/or drugs.

14. How has the exacerbation of the patient's illness affected her sleep patterns?

15. Evaluate Jacquline Catanazaro's participation in her care at the time of her illness.
    a. Active
    b. Moderately active
    c. Passive

16. What are Jacquline Catanazaro's primary concerns about being admitted to the hospital?
    a. Fear of losing independence
    b. Financial responsibility for hospital bills
    c. Fear of being poisoned by the medications prescribed
    d. Inability to be discharged in a timely manner

- Click on **Return to Nurses' Station**.
- Click on **MAR** and then on tab **402**.

17. _____ has been prescribed to manage Jacquline Catanazaro's schizophrenia.

18. With regard to the medication in the previous question, what nursing assessments should be completed for Jacquline Catanazaro?

19. Which of Jacquline Catanazaro's blood levels should be assessed before beginning therapy with the medication identified in question 17?